MW01612594

Stretch Therapy

A Comprehensive Guide to Basic Stretching

Emily A. Smith

Disclaimer: The information contained in this publication is provided on a strictly "as is" basis. The author of this publication makes no representations or warranties, express or implied, with respect to the contents or use of this publication, or any part thereof, and specifically disclaims any express or implied warranties or usefulness for any particular purpose of this publication. The author reserves the right to change or revise this publication, at any time.

Copyright ©2007 Emily A. Smith. All rights reserved. Neither this publication nor any part thereof may be reproduced, photocopied, storied in a retrieval system, or transmitted without the express prior consent of Emily A. Smith.

ISBN 978-1-4357-0348-3

Medical Advice: The author of this publication is not a medical Doctor. Nothing in this publication should be construed as an attempt to offer or render a medical opinion or otherwise engage in the practice of medicine. The medical information provided in this publication is, at best, of a general nature and cannot substitute for the advice of a medical professional. You are urged to consult with a qualified physician regarding personal health questions and conditions. Never disregard professional medical advice or delay in seeking it because of something you have read in this publication.

Foreword

The seeds of this book were planted in a session with a marathon runner. He had been a runner for almost twenty years and for the last thirteen weeks he had been out with a hamstring injury. He called me up and told me that some of his training friends had suggested that he come see me. I worked on him for an hour and a half and sent him home with some stretches to do daily. The following weekend, he ran his first race in over three months. He came in to see me after the race and said to me, "the difference between you and other therapists is that the stretches you gave me were so basic that I actually did them!" I jokingly said back to him, "I should write a book!" and the rest is in the following pages.

As a yoga instructor and former gymnast, I take for granted that stretching comes easily for me. I realize that yoga is not for everybody, HOWEVER...stretching is! As a clinical massage therapist I see many different people in my practice. Every time I work on these people, I give them certain stretches to do for whatever body part may be suffering from extreme tension. The clients who begin to practice these stretches always come back feeling much better. The ones who don't use them tend to maintain their tightness. While this may keep me in business, I would much rather see everyone using the stretches to better their lifestyle or performance! I decided to compile basic stretches for each body part so that you may always have them to look up and use at any time. It is with gratitude and love that I share them with you. May you use them as often as possible.

Table of Contents

Breathing:

Breathing is essential, we all know that. It is really important to use proper breathing while stretching. By doing so, you can largely increase the stretch. The best way to breathe while stretching, in my opinion, is to breathe through the nostrils for both the inhale and the exhale. Take slow, fluid, calm breaths using the navel as your guide. Inhale, let the navel expand away from your spine and exhale bringing the navel back toward the spine. An ideal amount of breath in a stretch would be inhale for a count of four and exhale for a count of eight. Try to keep the breath silent - the louder you breathe, the more stressful it is on the body and the breath tends to be more in the chest. You don't want your shoulders to rise up when you breathe in. Instead, the whole body stays relaxed and the navel and stomach move.

Use your breathing to increase the stretch by using the exhale to bring more heat to the muscle allowing them to stretch further. Inhale keeping the body still, exhale increasing the stretch slightly. When stretching, it is important to hold each stretch for at least twenty seconds to increase range of motion. A good rule for doing this would be five rounds of deep breaths over a period of about twenty seconds.

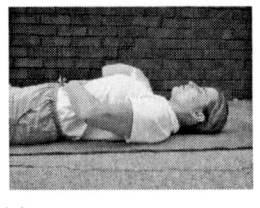 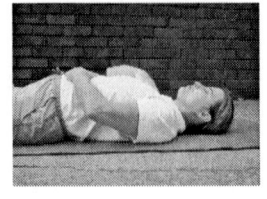 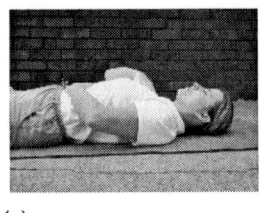

(a) (b) (c)

One way to practice relaxation breathing is to lie down flat on your back and place one hand on your stomach and one hand on your chest (a). When you inhale, the hand on the stomach rises up and the hand on your chest stays relaxed (b). Exhale and the hand on the stomach comes back down and again the hand on the chest hasn't moved (c). This way you can tell if you are relaxed when you're breathing and it's a wonderful, simple way to monitor your breathing.

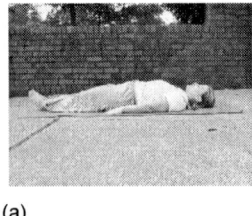 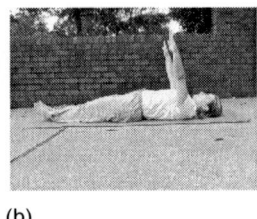 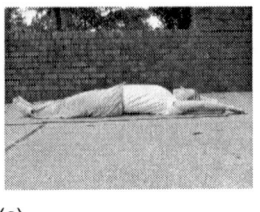

(a) (b) (c)

2) This exercise utilizes your entire lung capacity.The diaphragm is responsible for eighty percent of your breathing, while the sternum is responsible for ten percent and the collarbones take the other ten percent. Lying on your back with your legs extended, place your palms flat on the ground to your sides (a). On an inhale, lift your arms straight up (b) and back to a stretched position with the arms by your ears (c). On the exhale, bring the arms back down to your sides. The arms stay straight and they move at the speed of your breath. As the arms begin lifting, you can feel the diaphragm expanding (the belly). As the arms come over the chest, you can feel the chest taking part in the breath. As your arms are past your chest, you can feel the collarbones finishing the breath and the stretch. It is a very easy way to practice full breaths. This is nice to do when you get up in the morning before you get out of bed, and at night before you go to sleep.

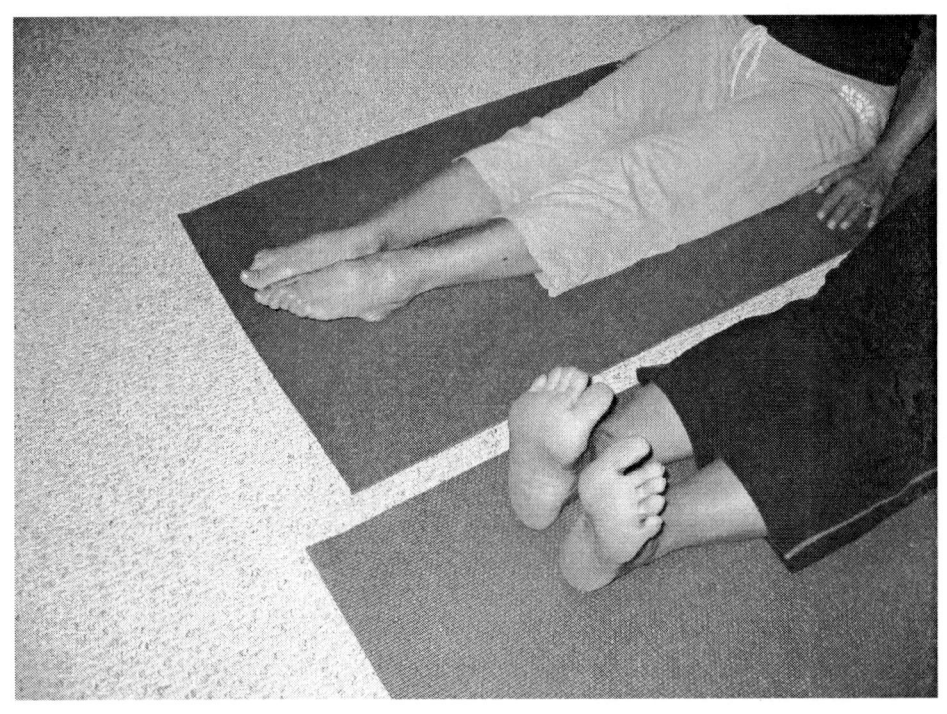

Wrist/Fingers/Ankles

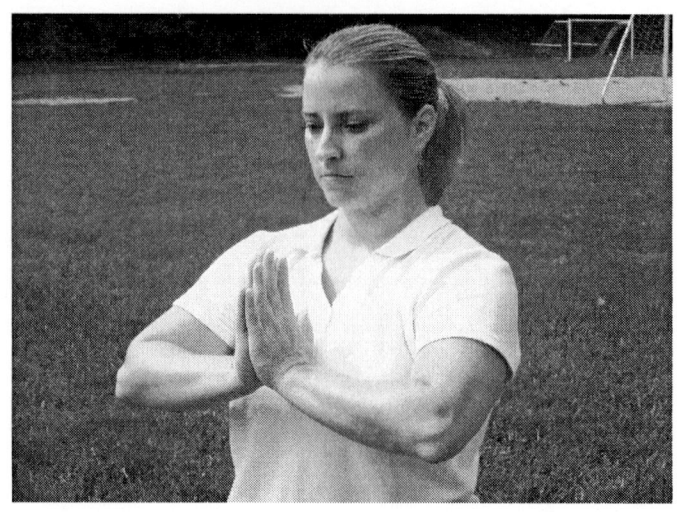

1) This simple wrist stretch can be done in virtually any body position; standing, seated, or walking. Simply place the palms of your hands together and try to relax the elbows. If you work with computers, practice this stretch hourly!

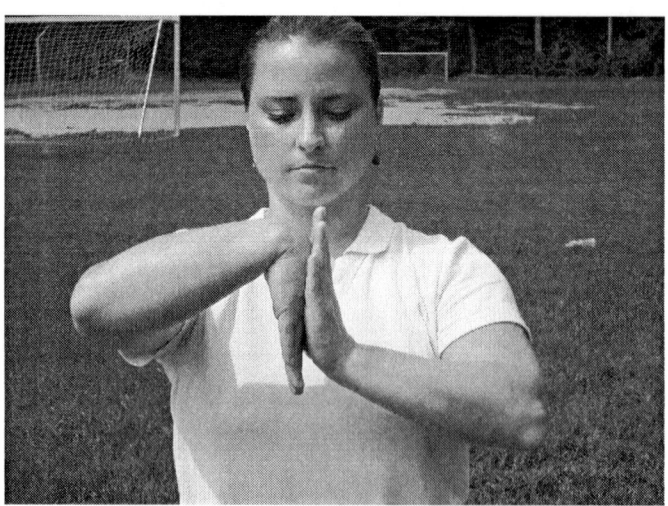

2) This is a variation of the previous stretch. Starting with the fingers up, palms facing each other, turn one hand fingers down so that one palm will be touching one knuckle side of the other hand. Keep both hands flat and relax the elbows.

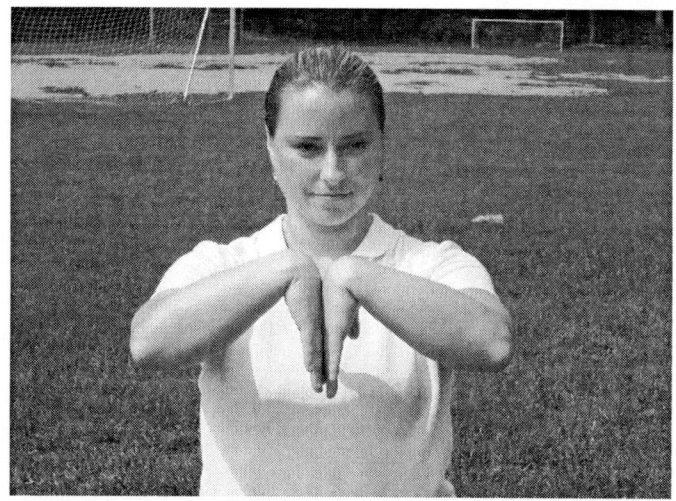

3) Place the knuckle side of both palms flat together and drop the elbows. If the elbows cannot drop below the plane of the wrists, this could be an indication of carpal tunnel syndrome. If this is the case, seek a good massage therapist or acupuncturist to help remedy this situation. Practice this entire wrist sequence often. If possible, do this many times throughout the day.

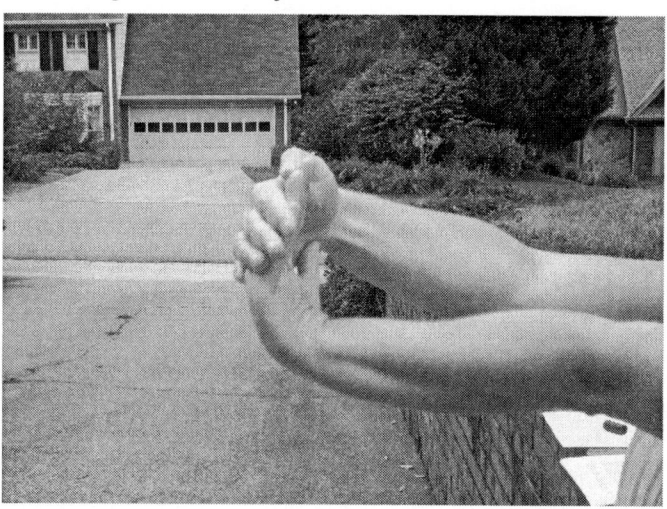

4) Extend one arm, palm out and fingers up. The knuckles are facing you and the palm of the hand faces out, away from the body. Place your other hand over the palm and the fingers, covering both areas so you're not pulling just your fingers back. The hand pulls the palm/fingers back toward your face. This stretches the wrist, the fingers and the forearms (the flexors).

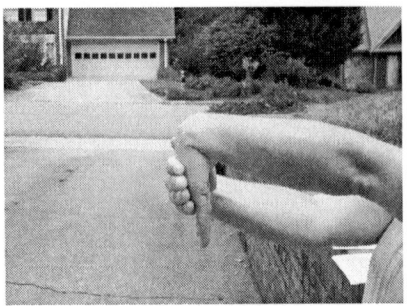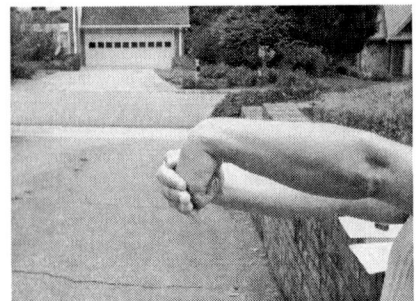

5) Turn the palm facing down so your finger tips face the ground. Place the other hand over the knuckles and fingers, and pull in toward your body. This stretches the forearms, as well as the wrists, and the fingers. Another option with this exact same stretch is to place your hand in a fist and the other hand pulls the fist down toward you. This adds to the stretch of the forearm (the extensors).

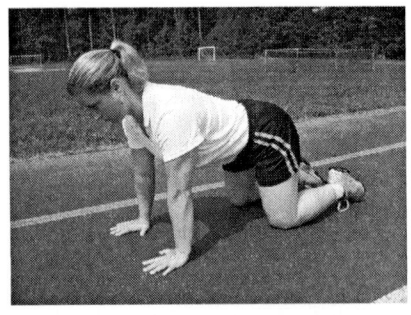
(a)
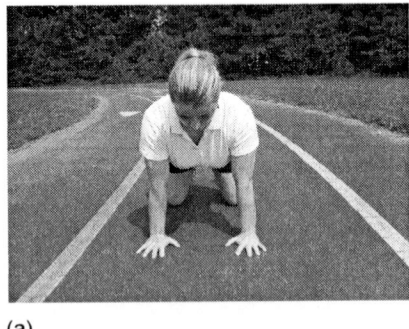
(a)

6) On your hands and knees, place the knees hip width apart and the palms of the hands directly underneath the chest, flat on the ground (a). The hands should be parallel to each other and flat. Keep the middle fingers on both hands facing forward as a guide.

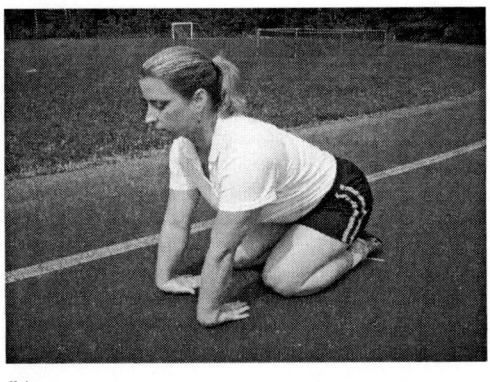

(b)

Now, turn your palms upward, keeping the fingertips facing your body (b). The knuckles are now on the ground and your palms face up. This time, sit back toward your heels, or on your heels. An option is to have your hands closer to your knees for this stretch.

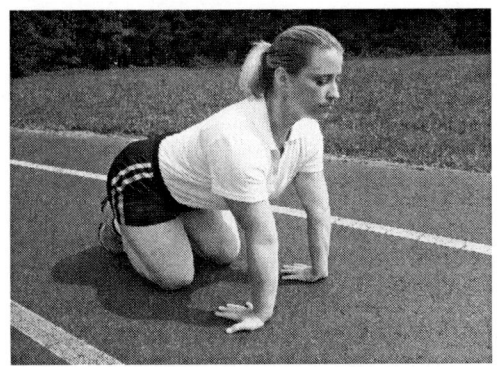

(c)

Place your palms flat on the ground, and your middle fingers face in toward your knees (c). So, the fingers face inward, the knuckles face up, and the palms are on the ground. As with the last stretch, lean back toward your heels for this stretch if it's comfortable.

Hold each of these wrist stretches a minimum of five deep breaths. In this time of computers and cell phones, it is extremely important to keep flexibility in your wrists and hands.

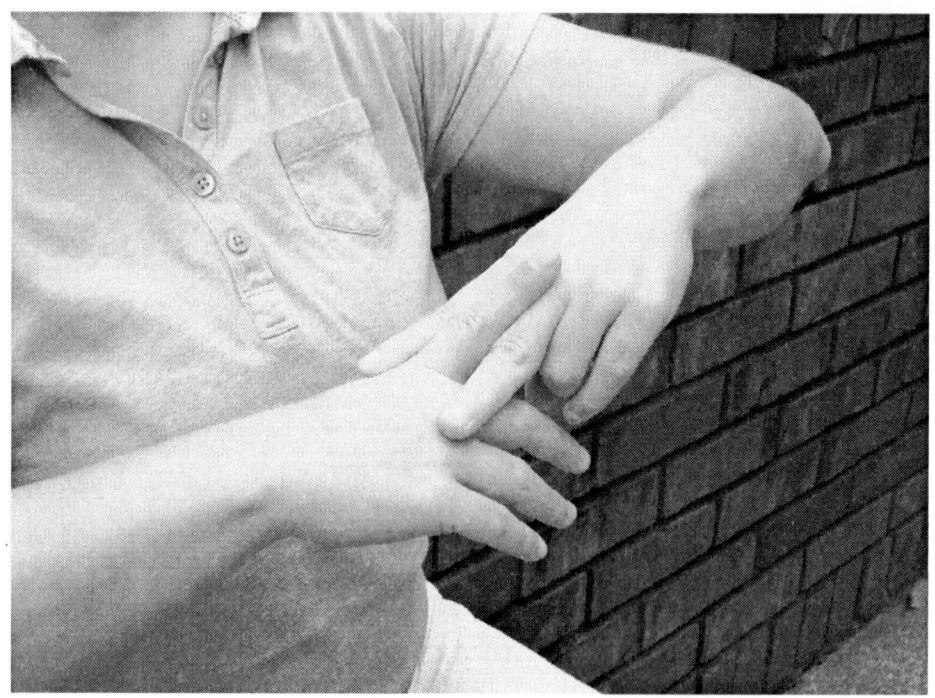

Fingers

This is an easy stretch for the fingers. If you play music, work on computers, write, etc., you use your fingers all the time. We tend to take for granted that the fingers need stretching. This stretch I learned from my reflexology teacher, and it has been very helpful for me.

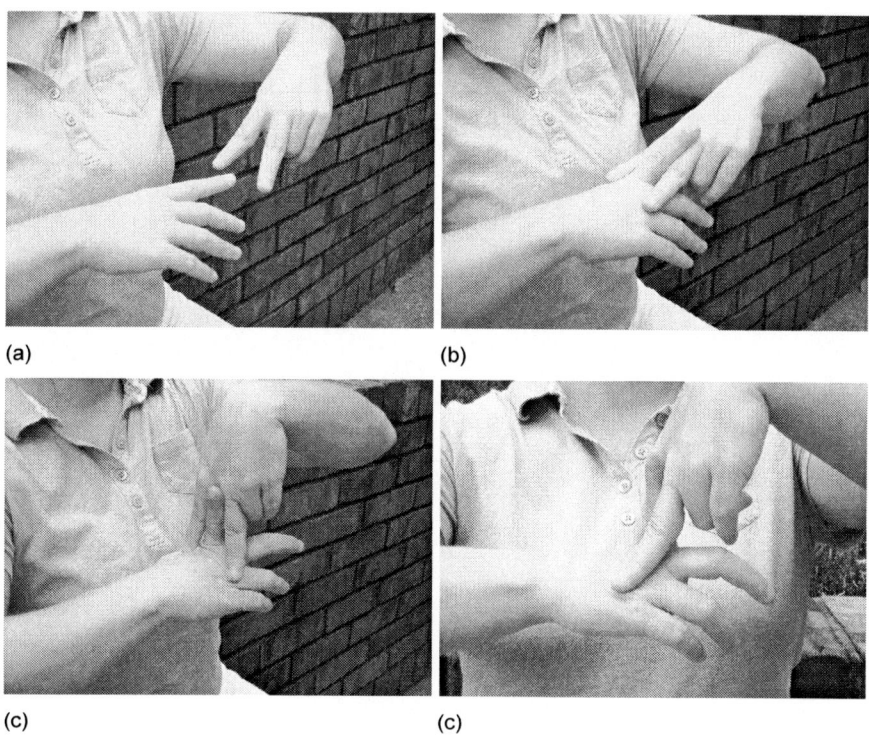

(a)   (b)

(c)   (c)

(1) Start with stretching the fingers on the right hand. The right hand is simply relaxed. To do this stretch you will use your index and middle fingers of the left hand. The index and middle fingers will form a V shape (a) to pick up a finger on the right hand and place the finger in the middle of the two fingers (b). Then lift your wrist up on your left hand to straighten the index finger and stretch it back (c). Hold this stretch for five deep breaths or more, and then move on to the next finger to stretch. From index to the pinky and then with your thumb. Then, do this to the other hand. Practice this stretch often and make sure you stretch every finger and not just the ones that you use most.

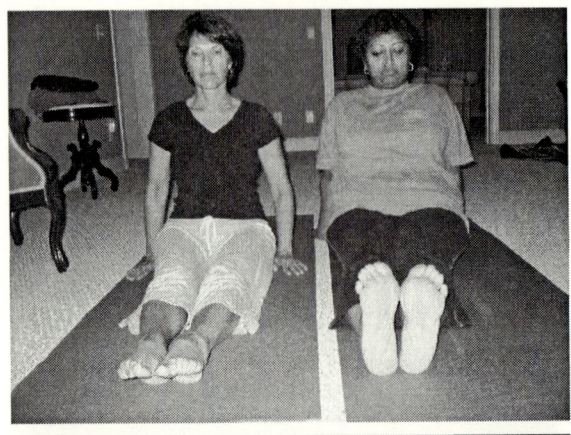

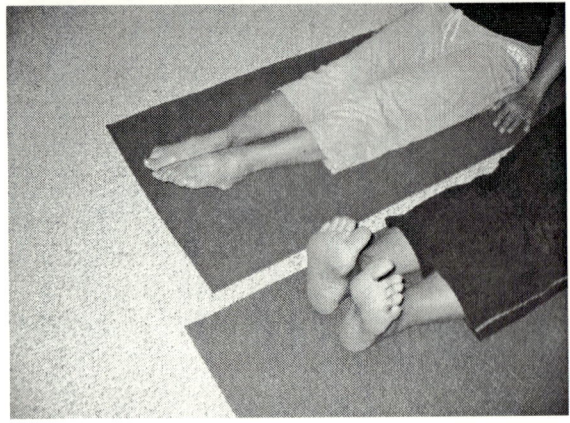

1) A simple, yet effective, way to keep the ankles loose is to point and flex your feet. Although it is simple and most people know this, we do not seem to put it into practice unless our ankles are bothering us! Let's think preventive here and do these stretches after every workout.

It's best or most comfortably done without shoes. Sit on the ground or lie down. Point the toes down toward the floor. This increases the arch in your foot and stretches the ankles.

2) Flex the foot by lifting the toes upward and trying to get the toes to face your head. This stretches the plantar fascia in the arch of the foot. If you are in a good flexed position, the heels will lift off the floor. Continue to point and flex the feet a few times, hold each stretch for at least two-three deep breaths. It's nice sometimes to add foot circles along with this, if you'd like.

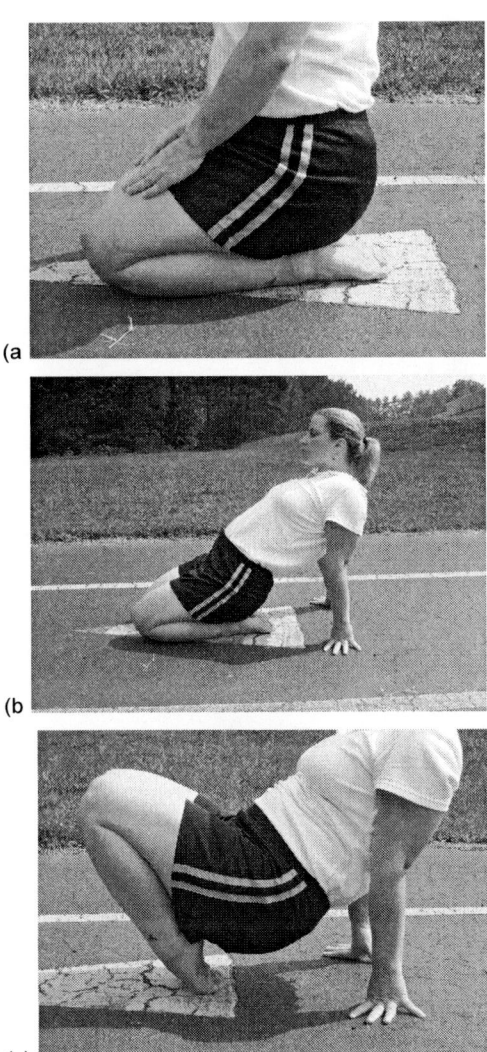

(a

(b

(c)

3) This stretch is much more difficult, but it really does the job! If you're a runner, you will not love this stretch, but your ankles will love you for doing it! Start by sitting on your heels (a). Keep your big toes touching, your heels touching, and your knees touching. First, place your hands behind you, as far as you can get them (b). Then, slowly roll back onto your toes (keep the toes curled under) and lift your knees up as high as you can get them (c). At first you will want to bail out of this stretch really quickly, but try your best to hold this stretch for at least three deep breaths. Immediately follow with the next stretch.

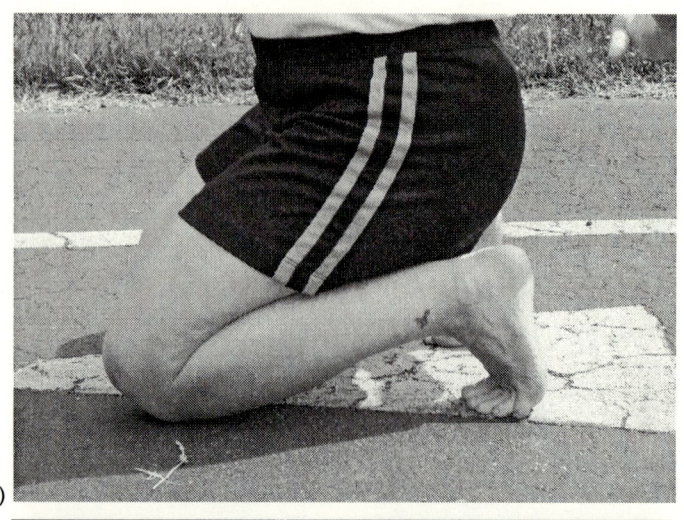

(a)

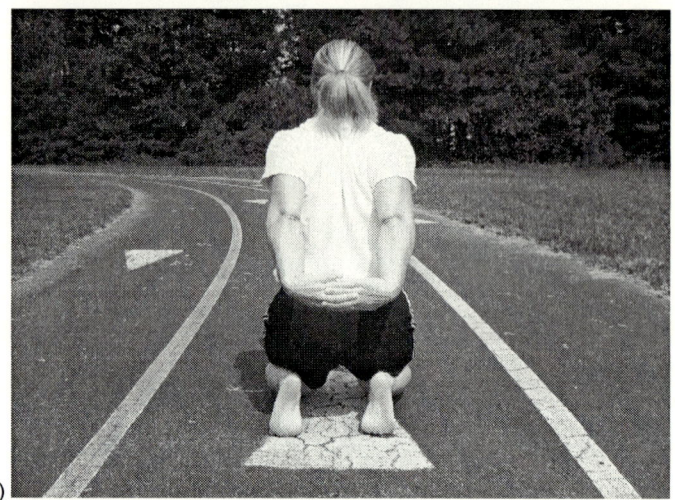

(a)

4) This time, tuck the toes and pads of the feet on the ground. The toes and pads should be completely flat on the ground and your heels face up, as you sit on your heels (a). This stretch is wonderful if you wear high heels often. To add to this stretch (and to take your mind off of the stretch) you can add a chest stretch by clasping your palms together behind your back and lifting the arms up. When I come out of this stretch I gently tap the tops of my feet on the ground a few times like making thunder sounds. This makes it easier to come out of these stretches. Stretch 3 and 4 are hard stretches, and as a result are usually not practiced often. However, if you have issues with your ankles and feet I would recommend making the effort to do these stretches, if it's not too painful. They are really incredible stretches.

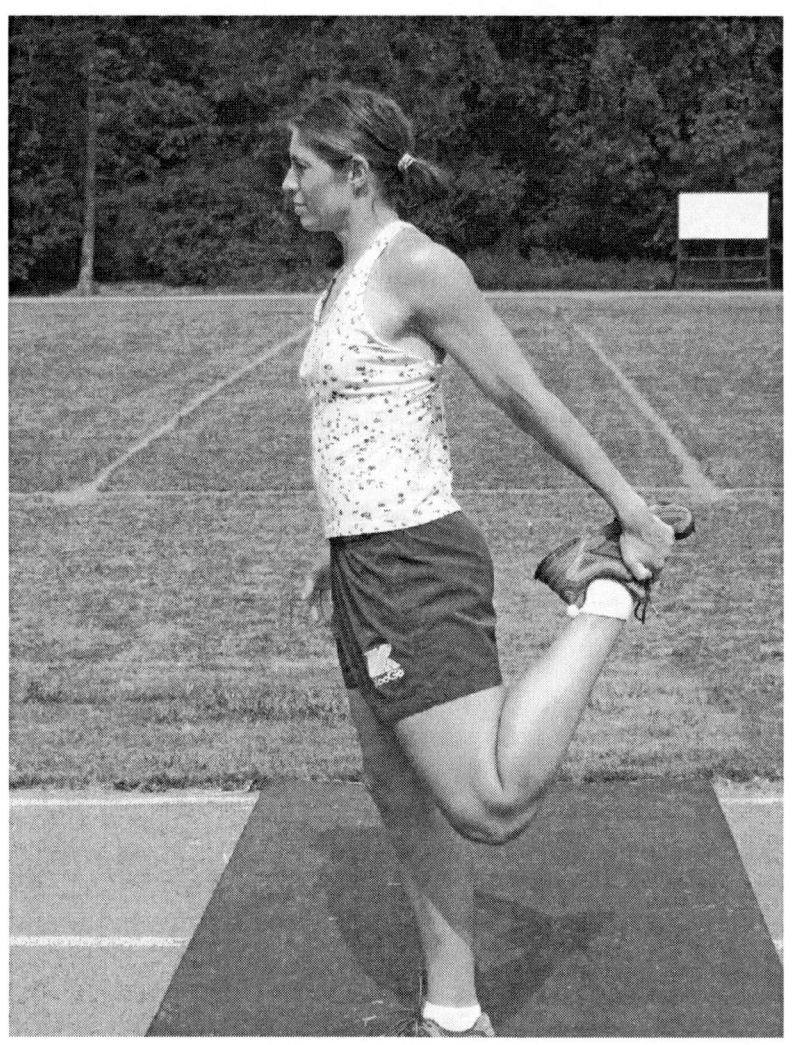

Legs

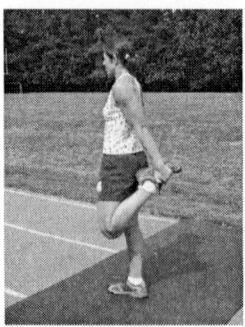

1) Standing on one leg and bending the other, hold the bent leg's foot in you hand. You want the heel to touch your buttocks for a good Quad stretch. If it's hard to hold your balance, hold on to something with the free hand. Hold this stretch keeping the base leg as straight as possible, bent leg parallel with base leg, keeping the back straight and head neutral.

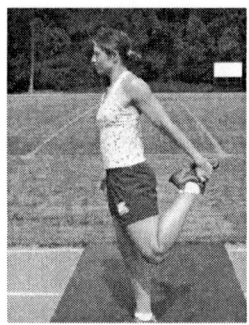

2) To increase this stretch and bring the stretch up into the hip flexors, the heel will actually not be touching the buttocks. The heel will be brought back slightly, but it will feel like a tug of war.

Push your heel against your hand. At the same time, gently try to pull your heel to your buttocks. You will create a gentle push-pull scenario. You will feel the stretch move higher than the leg and into the hip flexors (mainly the psoas which can be felt between the hip bone and the pubic bone). Again, keep the base leg straight, the spine straight and the head neutral. This is a small shift in movement, but it will make a big difference in the stretch.

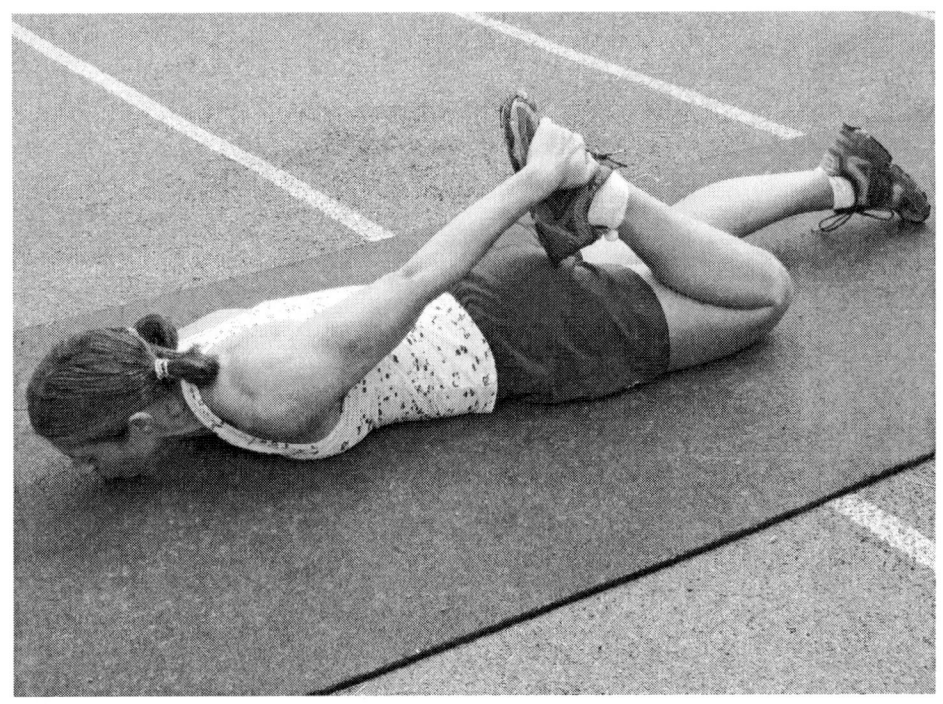

3) Lie down flat on your stomach and place your chin on the floor. If that is uncomfortable, you can turn your head to one side or the other. Keep one leg straight and bend the other knee, placing the foot in the hand. This is the same stretch as above but you are lying down this time. Pull the heel toward your bottom and hold this stretch. Breath slowly and deeply, and on the exhale, try to pull the heel a little bit closer to the buttocks.

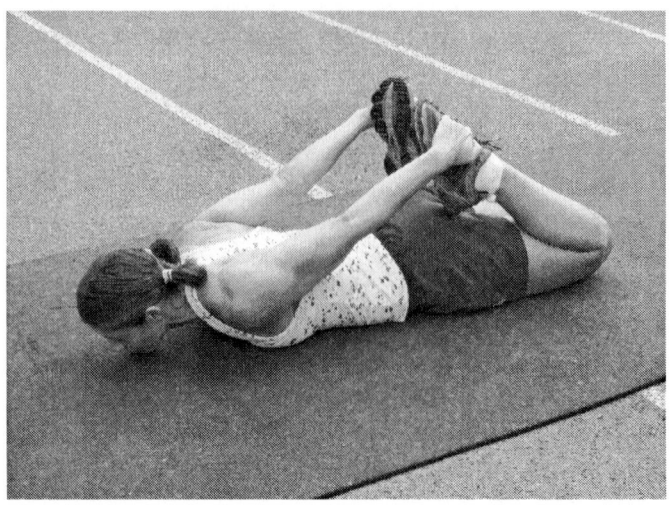

4) Bend both knees, placing feet in both hands (right foot in right hand and left foot in left hand). Pull both heels into the buttocks. Start this stretch with both knees on the ground and your chin on the ground.

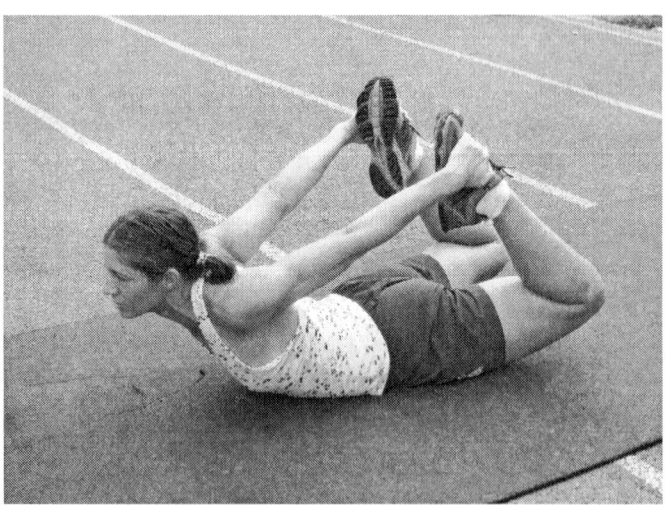

5) Slowly increase the stretch by lifting the chin up and trying to bring the knees up off the floor. When you are trying this stretch, think about stretching both the knees and the chin as far away from each other as possible. Slowly lift the chin up and the knees up at the same time. You want to allow the spine to stretch as well.

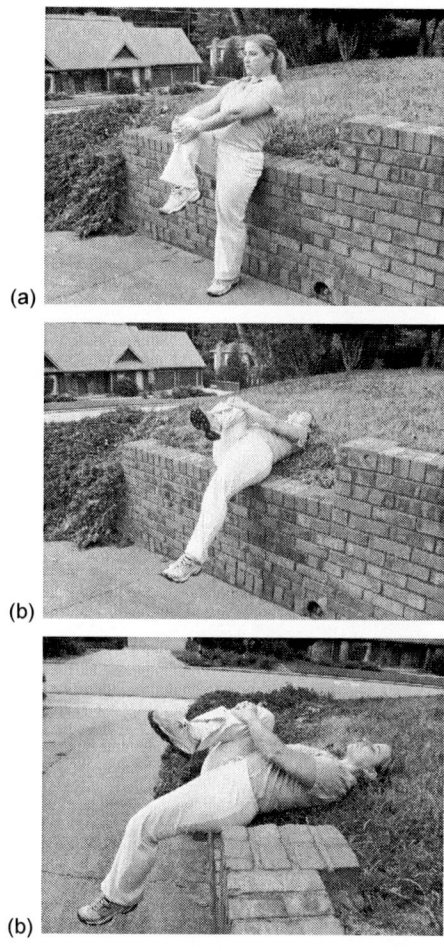

(a)

(b)

(b)

6) Psoas/Quad stretch. The psoas (or iliopsoas) muscle is the main hip flexor muscle located just above the quadriceps in the front hip area between the hipbone and pubic bone. This stretch is for the hip flexors and also for the quadriceps muscle that runs straight down the front of the leg (rectus femoris). This is done against the edge of the bed. (You can also do this in front of a table depending on the height of it.) Place your backside up against the edge of the bed. Hold one knee into the chest (a) and lie back onto the bed holding that knee (b). The stretch will be on the other leg. The leg that is not being held into the chest will drop down toward the floor. Keep your head on the bed, not up looking toward the leg, as it will decrease the stretch. Focus on really letting that extended leg stretch and lower toward the ground. Roll yourself back up and change sides. You should feel this in the upper part of the leg and hips.

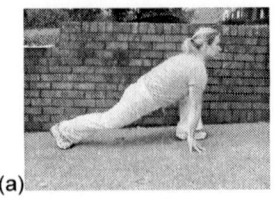
(a)

7) Come into a deep lunge position. Both feet are facing the same direction in a single line with the legs far apart. Square your hips to the front leg and bend your knee into a ninety-degree angle, placing the palms or fingertips on the ground on each side of the front foot (a). Keep your back leg straight. Push back toward your heel with the back leg and feel the stretch on the extended leg, in the quadriceps muscles.

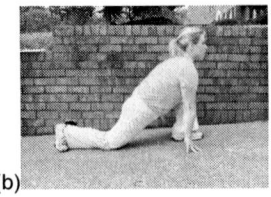
(b)

Continuing in the lunge position from the previous stretch, bend the back knee to the ground (b). Lift your chest up a little bit more and bring your body forward, letting the quadriceps and the hip flexors of the back leg stretch. Keep your fingertips or palms flat to the ground on each side of the front foot.

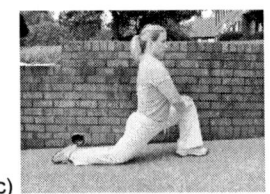
(c)

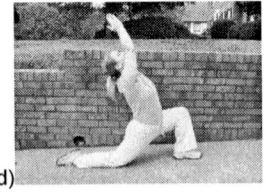
(d)

Start from the previous stretch, with the back knee on the ground. This time, place the top of your back foot flat on the ground. This will allow you to come even more forward with the front leg and chest. Lift your chest up and place your hands above the knee for balance (c). **Do not let your front knee go past the toes of your foot.** You can place your hands on your hips and lift the face and chest up for an increased stretch, or even more than that, you can lift your arms up overhead (d) and really feel the stretch through the quadriceps, hip flexors and stomach.

Hamstrings

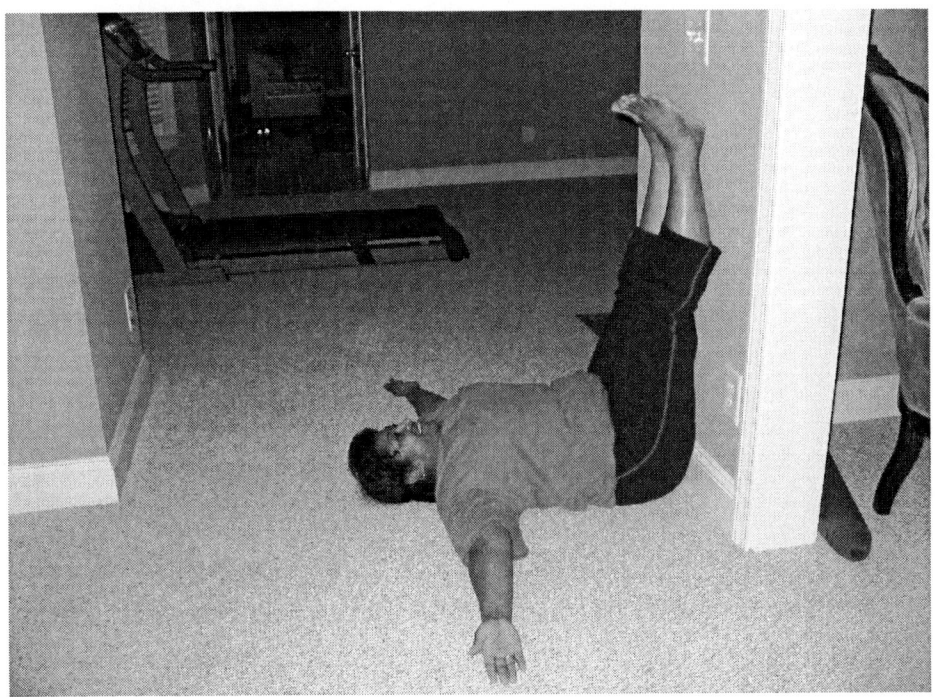

1) Let's start with a nice, easy hamstring stretch! This stretch is especially useful if you have extremely tight hamstrings, or have just suffered an injury to this muscle and need to start slow. Simply place both legs up on the wall. The trick is to keep the body in good alignment. Keep the legs straight, the hips squared to the legs, the back flat, the buttocks as close to the wall as you can get, and the neck straight. It feels good to keep the arms out to the side as well. The nice thing about this stretch is it's easy and you can hold it for a long time without tiring. I cannot stress how useful this simple stretch is. Do this stretch often!

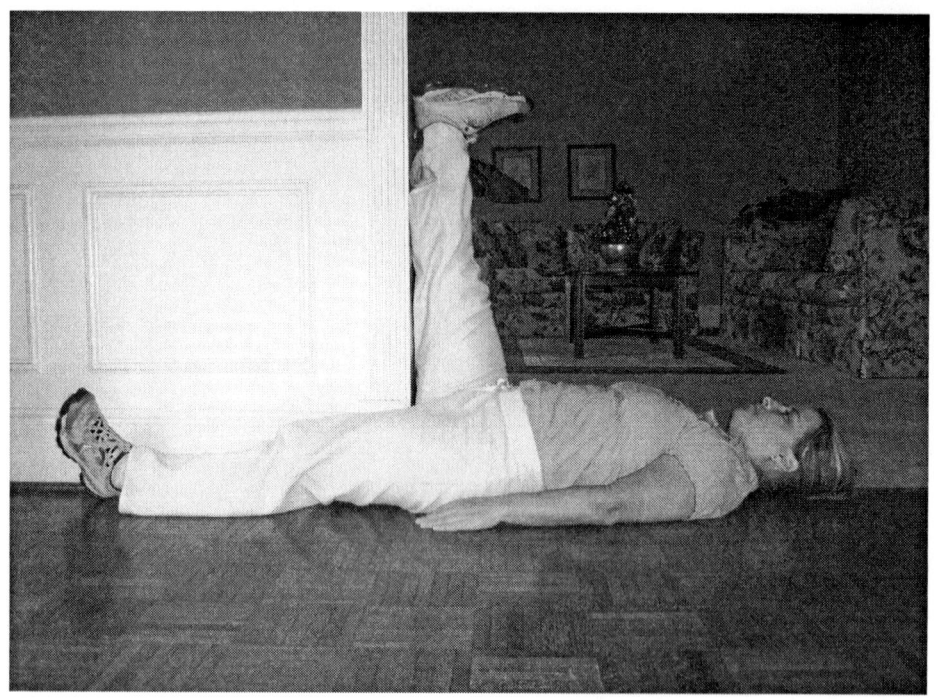

2) Another easier hamstring stretch involves a doorway. Lie down with your bottom against the doorway and slide one leg up the frame of the door. With the straight leg up against the doorway, allow the leg to rest on the frame of the door. The other leg is lying flat on the ground right next to the wall. Both legs are extended fully and the hamstring of the raised leg will stretch. It is important to keep your hips and low back flat to the floor. Hold this stretch more than the five breaths, as it is not hard on the body and relaxes the muscles nicely. Do this on both sides.

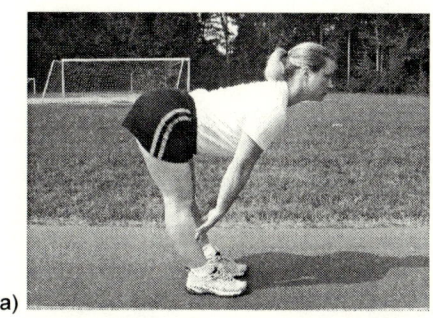

(a)

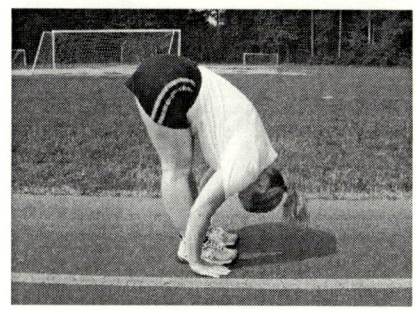

(b)

3) Place your feet hip width apart. Before you bend forward, extend the spine straight out and look up slightly. This will increase the stretch and allow the spine to bend more easily. Next, slowly bend at the hips, bringing your hands as close to the ground as possible. If you need to bend your knees slightly, you may do so, but ideally keep the legs as straight as possible for a better stretch. Relax the neck and let your head hang down without tension. Try to line your ears up with your arms as a way to check to make sure you are not looking up or holding the head. You want your hamstrings to loosen up, your back to be rounded and your neck to be relaxed. The more relaxed the other muscles can be, the easier it is to hold the stretch. Breath slowly and increase the stretch on the exhale.

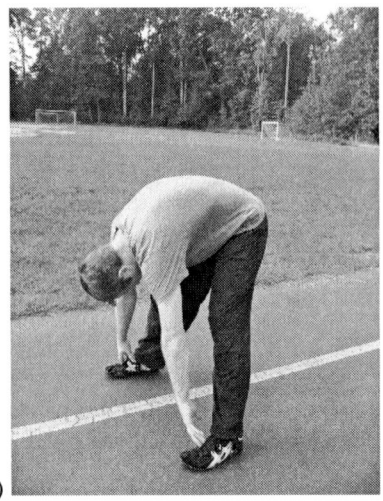
(a)

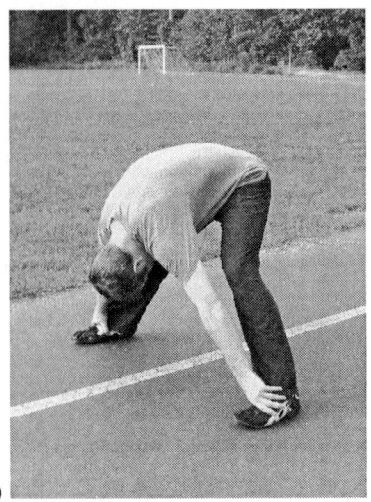
(a)

4) Spread the legs wider than hip width to a straddle stance. The feet are parallel, the hands reaching for the floor and the hanging down (a). If you need to bend the knees slightly it is fine, but try to keep the legs straight for best results.

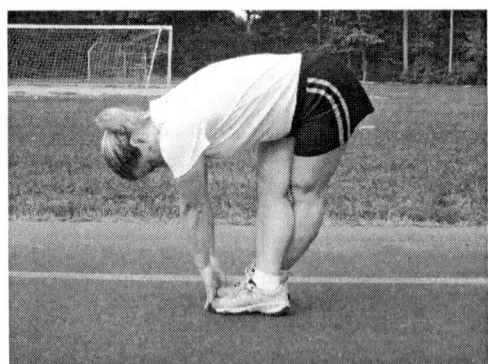

5) Cross one leg over the other and bend forward. This stretch adds the IT band (iliotibial band) as well as the hamstring. The IT band begins at the buttocks and comes down below the knee on the outside of the leg. Let your arms hang down and keep the neck relaxed. Change sides and repeat.

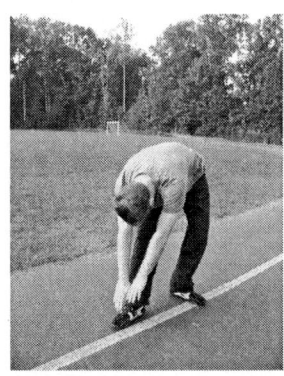

6) Stand with one leg back, the back knee is bent and the back foot is facing about forty-five degrees outward. The front leg is slightly bent but not as much as the back leg. The front leg is straight ahead and the foot faces front as well. Turn your hips toward the front leg and try to bring your hands to your foot. Place the foot flat on the ground and hold the foot. If both hands can't reach the foot, place one hand on the foot and one hand on your arm that's holding the foot. If neither hand can reach the foot, place your hands above the knee and continue to stretch forward.

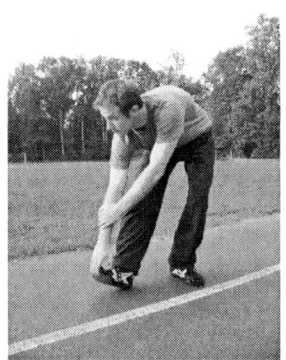

7) This is the exact same position as # 6 except you bring the front foot up-toes face up. This simply increases the stretch slightly. For this stretch, it is natural to lift the head up more than the other stretch. Whichever way is most comfortable for you is the way to do it, but keep the tension out of your neck.

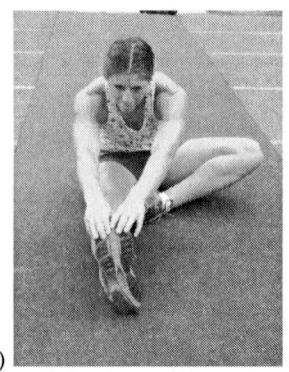
(a)

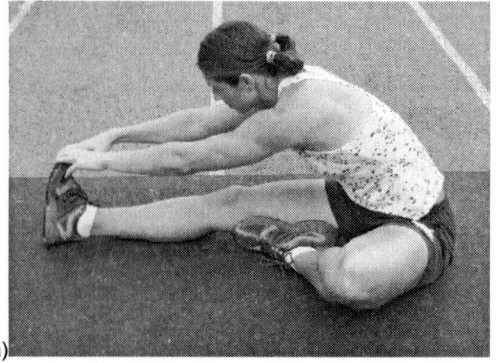
(a)

8) Sit on the ground, extend one leg out and bend the other knee, placing the heel into your inner thigh into the groin area (a). You want the extended leg as straight as possible and the bent knee to touch the ground, or as close to the ground as possible. The bent knee side stretches the adductors (inner thighs) and the straight leg stretches the hamstrings. Place both hands on the extended leg's foot or on the shin, if you can't yet reach the foot. Face both hipbones toward the straight leg. Before bending into this stretch, take a big inhale and lift your head and extend your spine. Then when you exhale, fold forward into the stretch. Again, keep the breathing slow and deep, and increase the stretch with each exhale. Come up from this stretch slowly, stacking the vertebrae of the spine by rounding up from the bottom to the top. Round your back as you come up and the head is the last to rise up. Change legs and repeat.

You can really increase this stretch by placing the heel of the bent leg on top of the thigh. Try to get the knee as close to the ground as possible. The top of the foot could be sitting in the fold of the hip. Round the ankle so that your foot is comfortable. Bend forward just as before, and come up just as before.

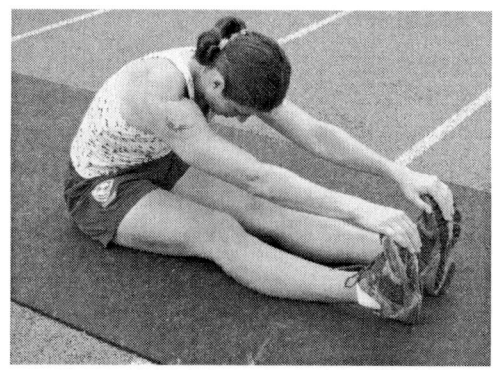

9) Sit on the ground with the legs extended and reach for your toes. Key points for this stretch are to keep the knees straight and keep the feet parallel to each other. Don't let the feet fall out to the sides when doing this stretch.

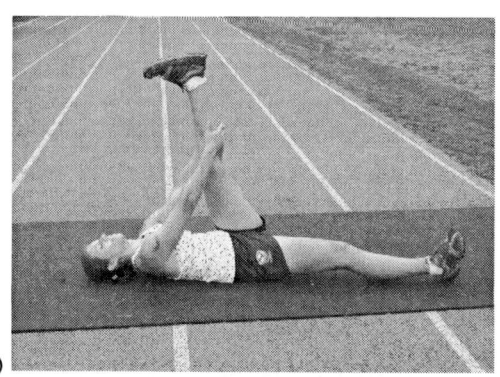

(a)

10) Lie flat on your back with your feet together, big toes touching and heels touching. Slowly lift one leg straight up into the air keeping the other leg straight on the ground. Try to push the knee of the straight leg down, keeping the leg straight (a). (Many people have a tendency to bend the lower leg to increase the stretch but it defeats the purpose. So, be extremely mindful of that lower leg-keep it down. If that means lightening the stretch on the extended leg, do so). Place the hands around the upper leg's calf. First, keep the head on the ground and just feel the stretch.

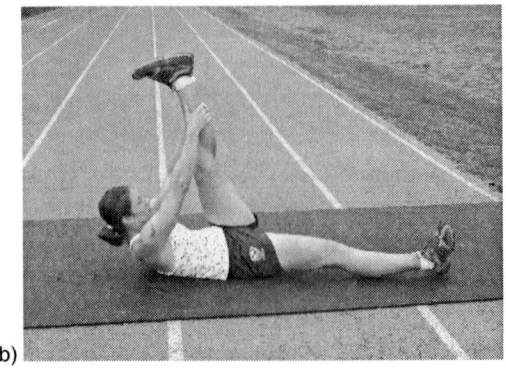

(b)

After about five deep breaths, on the next exhale, lift the head toward the knee and try to bring the leg closer to your head (b). Hold this stretch for at least five deep breaths. On each exhale, try to walk the hands higher up toward the ankle.

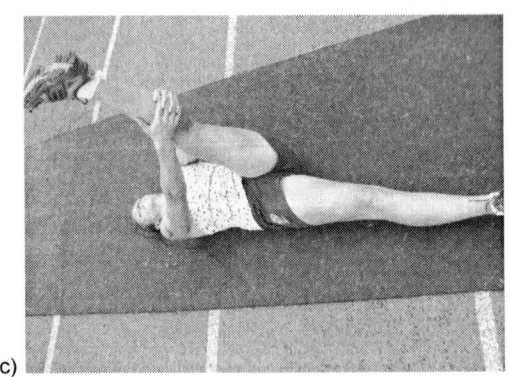

(c)

Then, lower the head again but keep the hands in their most recent position (c). Feel how the stretch has increased and hold this again to feel your range of motion increasing. This sequence can do wonders for the hamstrings, so try to practice this daily, especially after any exercise.

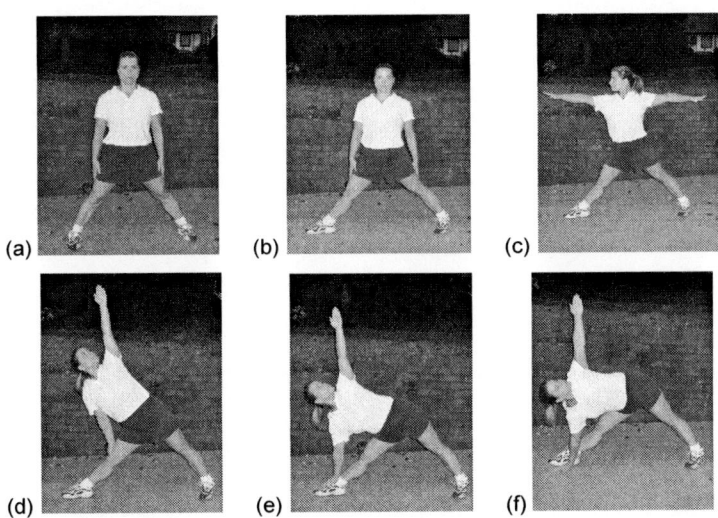

(a)　　　　　(b)　　　　　(c)

(d)　　　　　(e)　　　　　(f)

11) The "triangle" pose. Start with the feet wide and parallel (a). From parallel, the right foot rotates ninety degrees from straight out to the right (b). The left heel now inverts to a forty-five degree angle with the heel outward and the left toes turn in toward the direction of the right foot. Now, bring both arms out to the side at shoulder level (c). Look over the right foot as you inhale, lift the chest, and as you exhale, tip from the hips bringing your right hand down the right leg. The left arm is up by your left ear facing straight up to the ceiling (d). You have a few options for the right hand placement depending on your level of flexibility. First, you can place your right hand above your knee on the right leg and rest it there. If you can go further, you can reach your right shin, or try to place your palm on your right foot (e). If you can go even farther than that, place the palm of the right hand on the ground in front of your foot (f), still keeping the left arm extended and reaching up through that left side for balance and strength. Hold this stretch for at least five deep breaths and then slowly come up by tightening your stomach and change sides. The left foot now turns to ninety degrees and the right to forty-five and inverted, making sure the heel is facing out. It's common for people to have that back foot straight out instead of angled, but try to be mindful of this and push that heel out. Place your arms out to the side and bend to the left side, extending that right arm up to the sky and the left hand reaches for whatever level it wants and needs to feel the stretch in those hamstrings. This should also stretch the upper body, as your back should be flat and your chest should be open and stretching. If this pose is difficult for you, try doing this stretch against a wall, the back of the body and heels line up to the wall. It will help keep you in good alignment and is easier to balance.

Calves

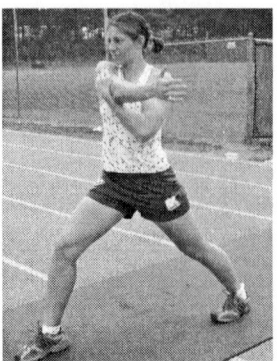

1) Stand in a lunge. Have both feet face forward. When the back heel is flat to the ground, you are stretching the gastrocnemius (the calve). Really push that back heel down flat and hold the stretch. To add an arm stretch (triceps), simply pull one arm across your chest and hold it with the other hand. Keep the hand off the elbow place the palm past your elbow toward the shoulder, or in front of the elbow on the forearm.

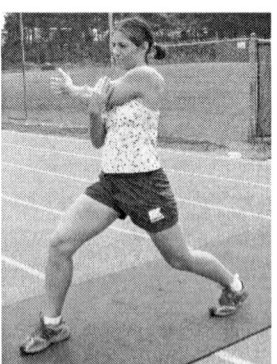

2) A variation of this stretch is to slightly bend the back knee. This adds another deeper calve stretch to a muscle that runs under the belly of the gastrocnemius called the soleus. It is important to stretch both the gastrocnemius and the soleus. Keep adding the arm stretches if you want, or keep your hands on your hips if it's easier for you.

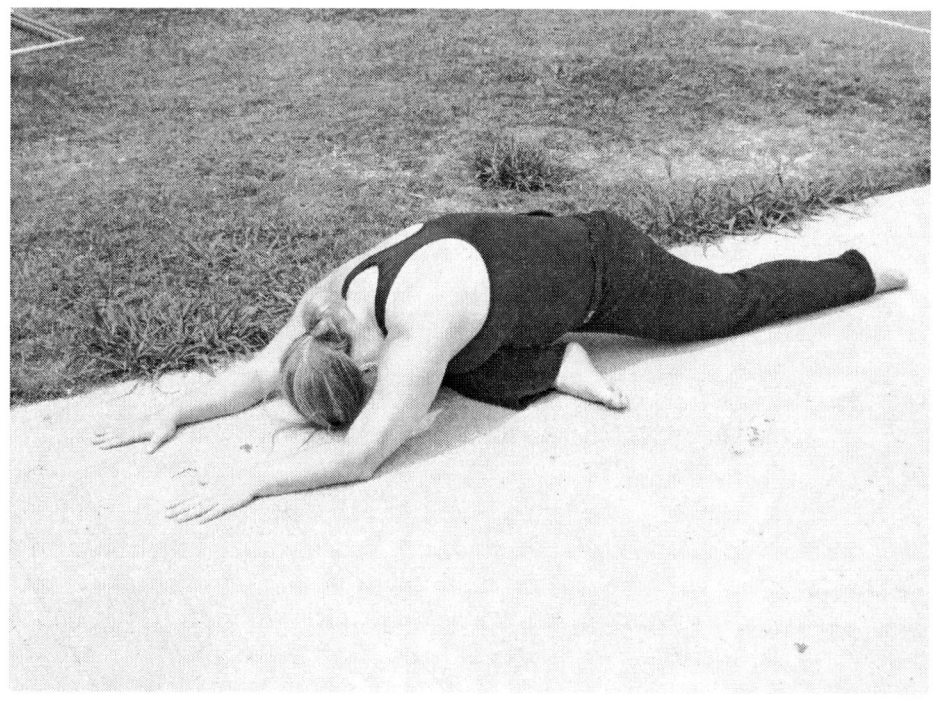

Hips/Buttocks

When I refer to the hips and buttocks there is one key muscle that I am trying to focus on called the piriformis. This small but important muscle is located from the upper middle part of the buttocks to the lower outer part of the buttocks and can cause a lot of problems if it's too tight. The sciatic nerve runs underneath this particular muscle and when this muscle gets too tight it can trap that nerve causing you sciatica like pain. It is imperative that we focus on this muscle group and practice these stretches often.

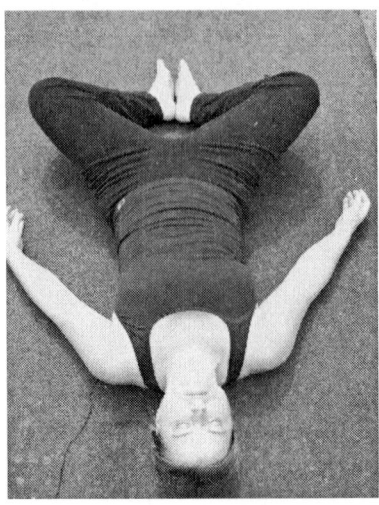

1) Lying flat on your back with your head straight and your arms in a relaxed position place the soles of your feet together and let the knees fall out to each side. This stretches the back, the hips and the adductors (inner thigh muscles).

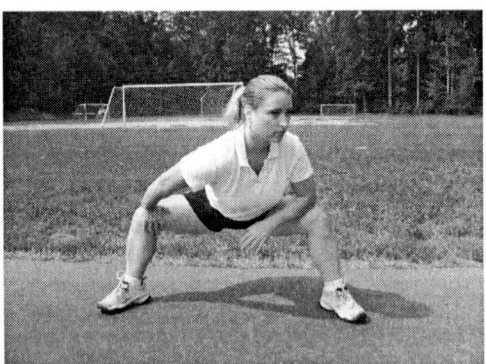

2) Stand with your legs in a wide stance with your feet parallel. Bend both knees and place the palms on the inside of each knee. To stretch the right side inner thigh (adductors) push with the right palm into the knee and look over the left side as shown. To stretch the left side, push with the left palm and look over the right side.

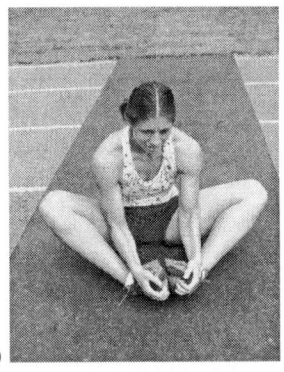 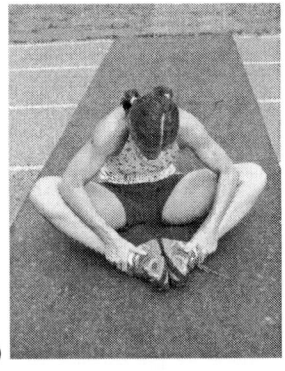

(a)   (b)

3) The "butterfly" stretch (as we call it in gymnastics). Sit on your bottom and place the soles of the feet together. First hold on to the feet and let the knees fall out to each side (a). Try to bring your head down to your feet (b) and hold at least five deep breaths. To increase the stretch it is really helpful to lift your head and chest up on the inhale and then bend forward on the exhale. If you find your knees to have difficulty relaxing, place the elbows on the insides of the knees and as you stretch downward, use the elbows to push the knees outward to increase the stretch for the adductors. Come up slowly, rounding the back, with your head as the last thing to come up. Breathe deeply.

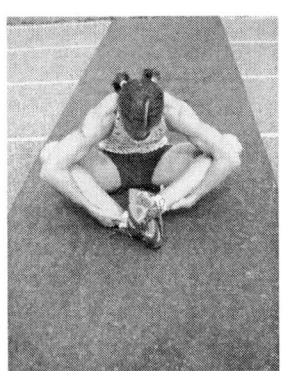

4) A modification to the previous stretch. Place one foot on top of the other foot as shown but remain in the "butterfly" position. Now fold forward and feel the difference on the outside of thigh (abductors) and piriformis. Return to seated position in the same way. When you come up, round the back and let the head be the last thing to come up and then change sides.

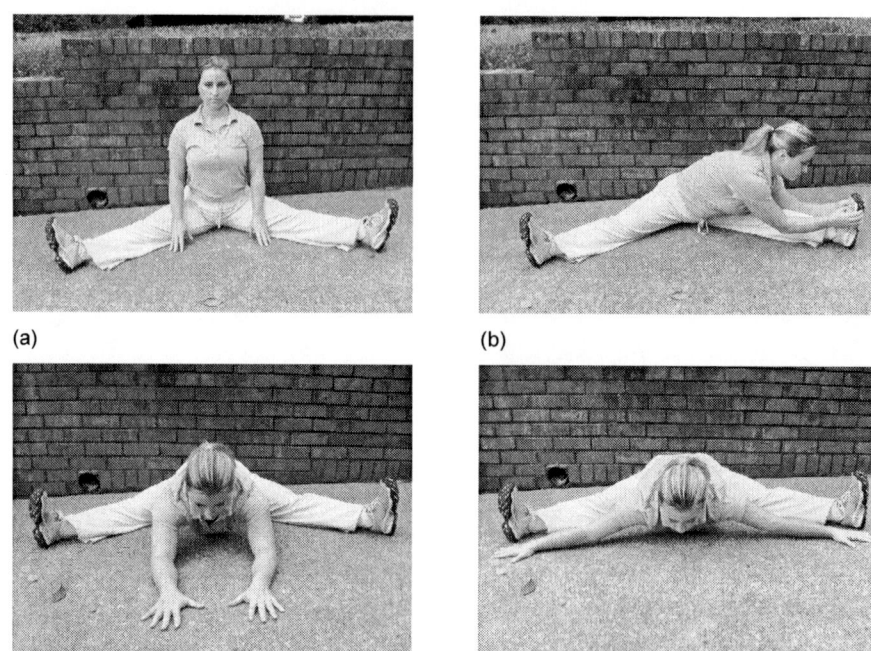

(a)

(b)

(c)

(d)

5) The "straddle" (as we also call it in gymnastics). Sit on your bottom and spread the legs out wide. Keep the knees and the feet facing up (a). You can walk your hands to one side and then the other (b) and then try to come down the middle (c). Try to extend your arms outward (d) or try to grab your legs with your arms. Breathe slowly and deeply and hold each of these positions before coming up. Do not bend your knees, as this cancels out the stretch and fires your hamstrings. You don't have to go flat like a pancake, just do what you can do in good form. If that means having the legs out and barely getting your hands to touch the floor, that's great! Your range will improve with practice.

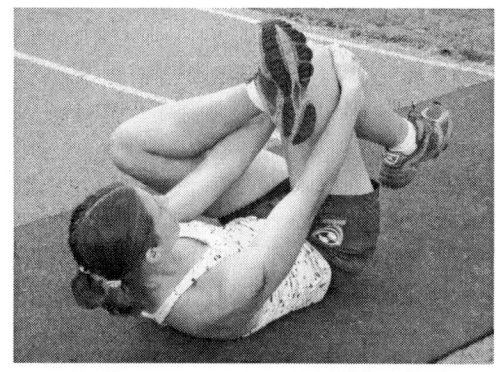
(a)

6) "Figure 4". Lie on your back and place both feet on the ground with both knees bent. Lift the left leg up and cross it over the right bent knee. Bring your left arm inside your left leg and your right arm outside your right leg and clasp your hands together (a). Lift the legs with your hands up toward the chest. You can lift your head up to increase the stretch.

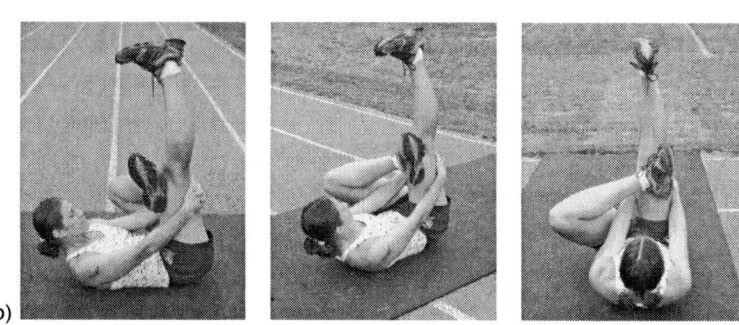
(b)

7) A variation of the Figure 4 is to simply straighten the top leg (b). In this example, it would be to straighten the right leg. This gives an additional hamstring stretch along with the hips and buttocks. Then change legs. Now the left leg will cross over the right bent leg and your left hand will come from inside and the right from the outside and connect the hands. Lift the knees to the chest and after a minimum of five deep breaths, switch to the left leg.

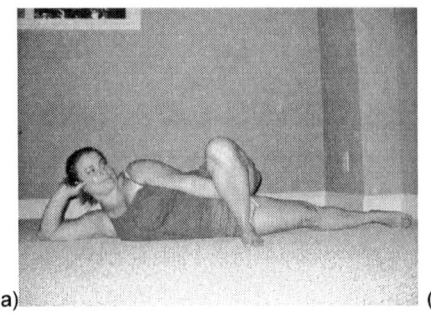
(a)
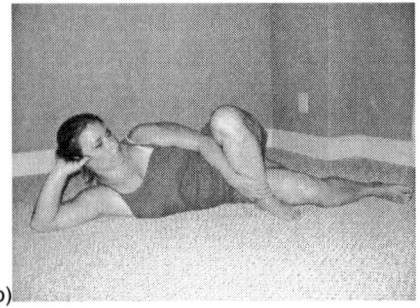
(b)

8) Lie on your side and rest your head on your hand. Bend the arm and bring the hand up to meet the head. Lie on your side. Bend your top knee and place that foot flat on the floor as high up toward your chest as possible (a). This stretches the piriformis and the abductors. Make sure your front foot is flat on the floor and try to get it higher than the bottom knee. To add on to this stretch, bend the bottom knee toward your chest. So, the right leg will now help the stretch of the already bent left side (b). Switch sides.

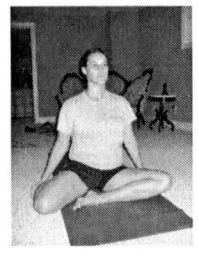
(a)
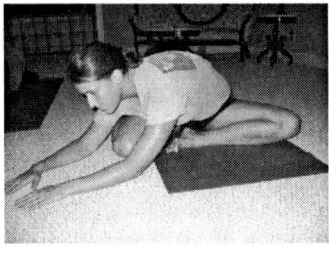
(b)
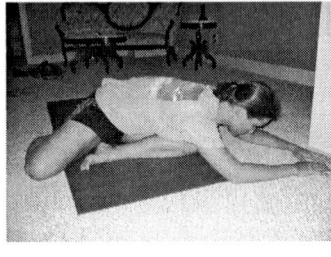
(c)

9) Sit on your bottom with one leg bent in front of you and one leg bent behind you. The foot of the leg behind you is facing the buttocks. Start with the left leg bent in front of you and the right leg bent behind you (a). First, turn to your right knee and try to bring both arms extended to or past that right knee (b). Hold for five deep breaths minimum and then come back up to seated. Then look at your left knee and face your center toward the left knee and walk your arms to or past the left knee (c). You can also stretch to the center of both knees by walking the arms straight out in front of you.

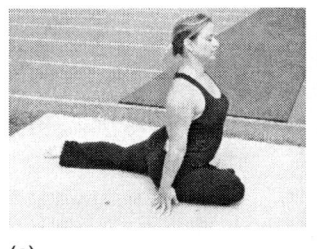
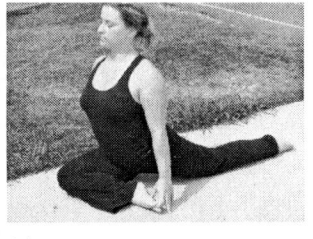
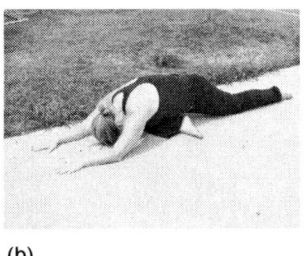

(a)   (a)   (b)

10) "The Pigeon." This stretch is the ultimate piriformis stretch. Practice this stretch often, and you will reduce your chances of sciatic pain. This is not, of course, a guarantee, but it is a good defense. Start with the front leg (we'll start with the right leg) bent in front of you as in the previous stretch. Then straighten your back leg. The left leg will extend behind you with the knee facing straight down to the ground (a). Bring your body weight to be centered over both hips. Don't lean on the bent knee side. Stay straight and centered. First, stretch your upper body upward with your hands on the ground on each side of your body. Then with a deep inhale, stretch the chest upward and on the exhale, walk your hands out in front of you (b). If you cannot extend your arms all the way out, that's okay, you can bend them and rest your head in your palms. Hold this stretch more than the minimum five deep breaths.

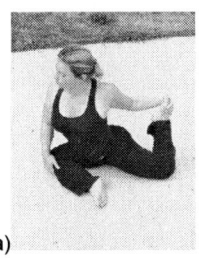
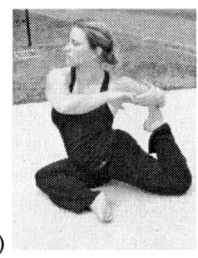
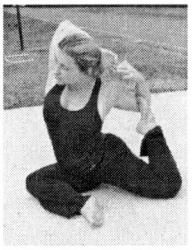

(a)   (b)   (c)

*11) The following are variations of the pigeon only to be done if you can sit in pigeon comfortably. The first is to come back up to the starting position. The legs do not change but the chest comes back up. Bend the back leg and hold the foot with the same hand (a). This gives you a big stretch in the quadriceps. To add to this, you may wrap your arm around your back leg and connect your hands together around the foot (b). Third, you can bring your opposite arm up over your head and grab the first hand. The foot is tucked into the crease of the arm (c). This gives you a piriformis stretch, a quadriceps stretch and a chest stretch. You are sitting balanced on the triangle of the front leg. When you're finished, change sides. You will more than likely find one side to be much looser than the other side.

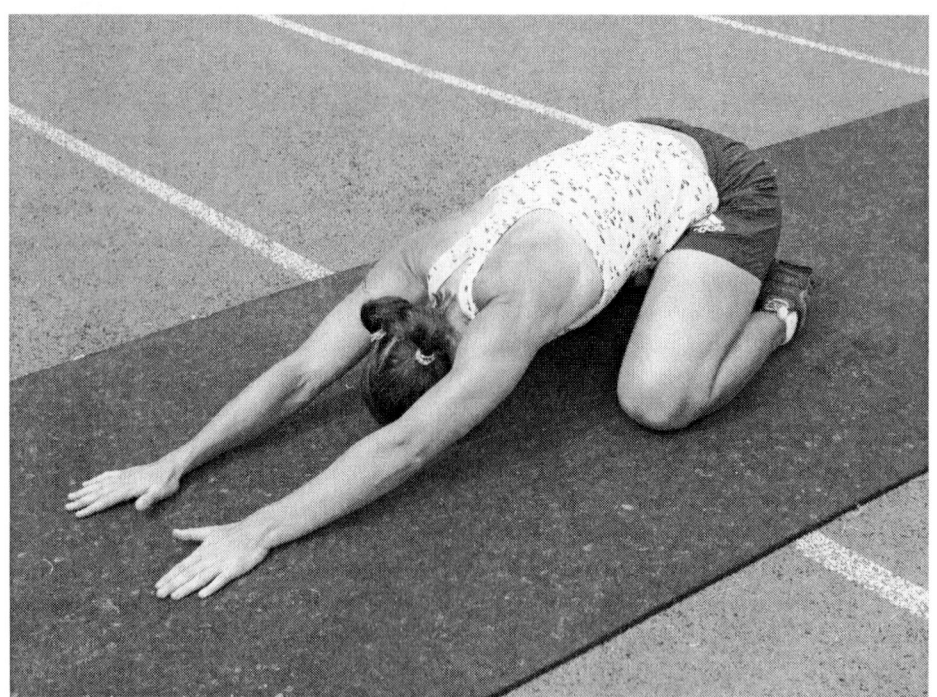

Back

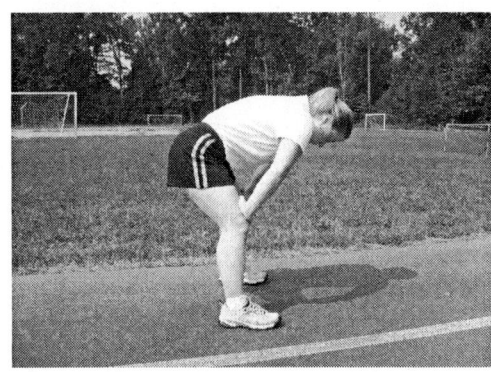

1) Standing in a wide stance with your feet parallel, place your palms on the insides of your knees. Slowly bend forward, rounding the back and dropping the head. Hold this position until you feel your back relaxing a bit-generally five deep breaths. Slowly round your back up, stacking the vertebrae from low back to neck. The head is the last thing to come up. Take a nice big inhale as the head lifts and then exhale when your head is sitting neutral.

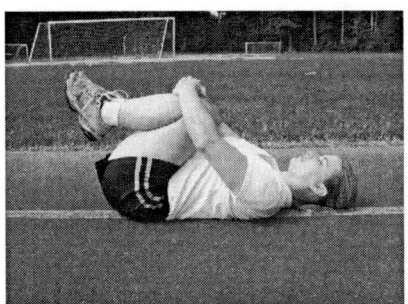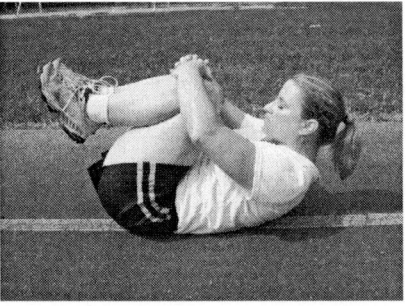

2) Lying down on your back, hug both knees into the chest. Take at least three to five deep breaths, and on an exhale, lift the head toward your knees. Think about trying to kiss your knees. Hold this position for another three to five deep breaths and then on an exhale, lower the head back down. Continue to hold the knees into the chest and relax the chin and neck.

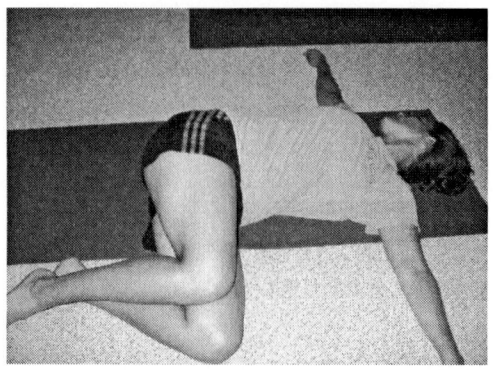

3) Keeping both knees bent, gently let both knees fall to one side. Keep your back as flat on the ground as possible and extend both arms flat to each side, or hold your knees with one hand and extend the other arm out. Example: If your legs are both to the right side, then hold the legs with the right hand, extend the left arm out to the side and look over your left shoulder to increase the stretch. It is important to keep the extended arm's shoulder/shoulder blade flat to the ground. This adds a nice chest and bicep stretch in addition to the back stretch and keeps the alignment appropriate in the back. Then roll the knees to the left, hold the knees with the left hand and extend the right arm out to the side looking over the right shoulder.

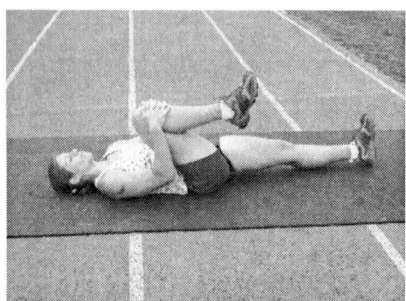
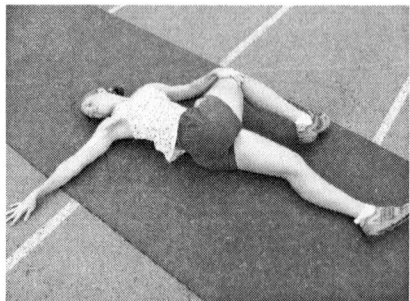

4) Come back to hugging both knees into the chest and then extend one leg straight out in front of you. Holding the right knee into the chest, the left leg is now straight. Then, roll the right knee to your left side. Hold the right knee with the left hand and extend the right arm out to the side looking over the right shoulder. This is like the previous stretch except this time it is only one leg that is bent. Hold at least five deep breaths and then hug your knees back to the center and release the right leg and hold the left knee into the chest. Turn to the right side now. Hold the left knee with the right hand and extend the left arm to the side, shoulder down and looking over the left shoulder. After at least five deep breaths come back to center and hug both knees.

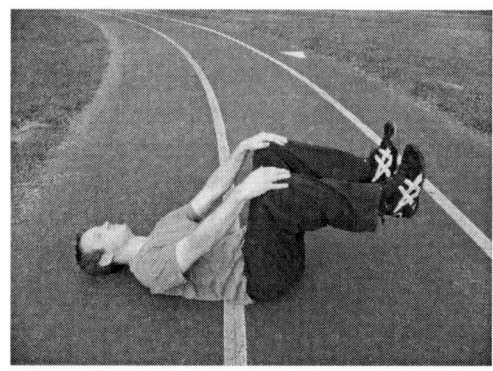

5) A modified stretch is to let the knees be over the hips more, instead of trying to pull them upward. Your knees are at a ninety-degree angle and your back is flat. Place your palms on the knees, or just below the knees and hold. Keep your head on the ground and simply let the back stretch. Breathe deeply and rhythmically. This is also great to do with your feet on a wall. You can let your arms fall out to the side, if your feet are supported by the wall.

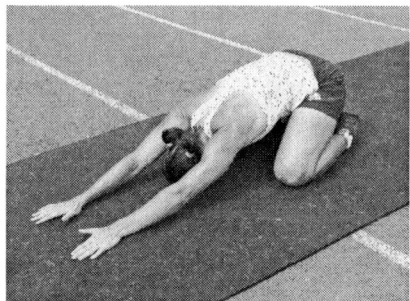 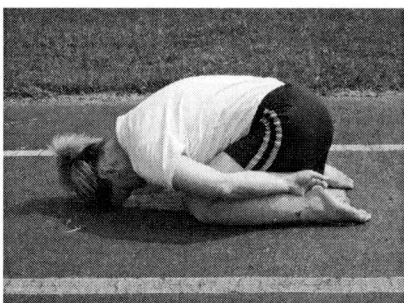

6) The "Child's Pose", as we call it in yoga. This one is for everyone-including of course, babies! In fact, they taught us how to do this stretch! Simply sit back on your heels and bring your head down to the ground. There are a few different arm positions, and it completely depends on your level of comfort. First, extend the arms out and use your hands to push your buttocks back onto the heels. A second arm position is called a modified child's pose with your palms facing up and your head resting in your hands. Keep the buttocks back on the heels, of course. Third, you can place your forehead down on the ground and bring your arms back behind you and hold your heels with your hands - or just let your hands lay on the ground by your heels.

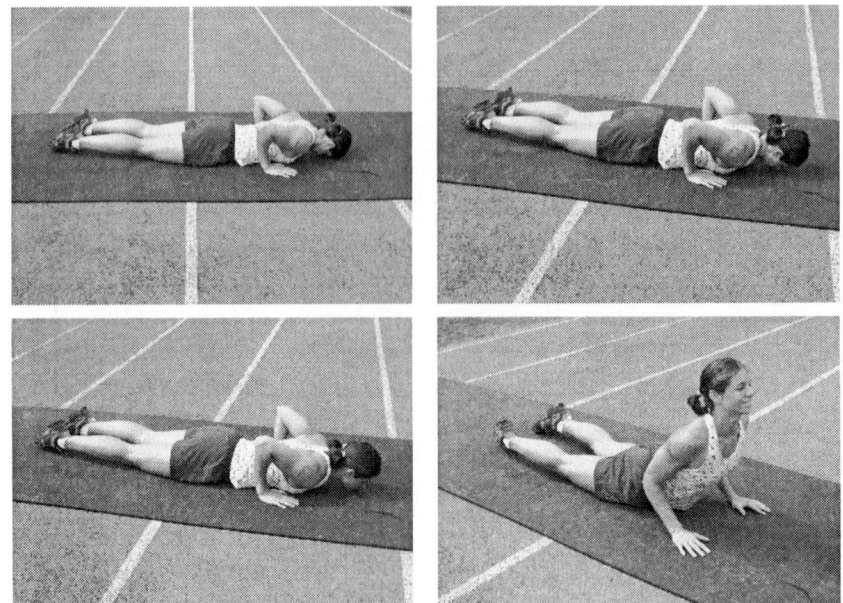

7) The "Cobra," as yogi's call it. This is not only an excellent stretch for the spine, but also for the stomach and chest. Start by lying flat on your stomach with your palms flat underneath the shoulders. The elbows face straight up to the ceiling and the tops of the feet are flat on the ground. Lift your head starting with touching the forehead to the ground, then touching the nose to the ground, then the chin touches the ground and as you lift the chin up, the upper body lifts as your head continues to look up and back. Come up high enough so that your chest opens up and try to touch your shoulder blades together in the back. Don't come up so high that you feel a strain in the back or chest. You want to stretch the muscles, but you don't want to overdo with this one. You are simply stretching your spine and chest. Hold for three to five deep breaths and then slowly roll yourself back down, starting with the chest, then the head ending with the forehead back on the ground.

* When you finish this stretch sit back into a child's pose for best results. It feels wonderful and is an excellent compliment to the movement you just did.

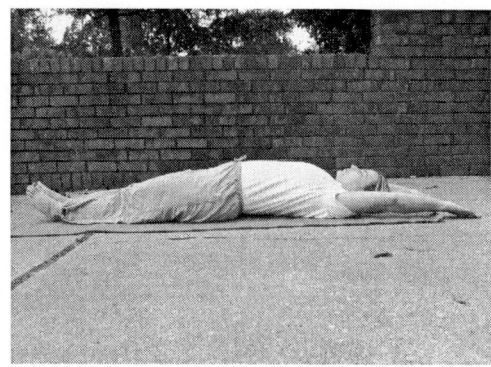

8) This is a simple, very nice whole body stretch, but the focus is stretching the spine. Lie flat on your back, extend the arms overhead and extend the heels away from your body. Keep the chin in and stretch the body as long as you can, from head to toe.

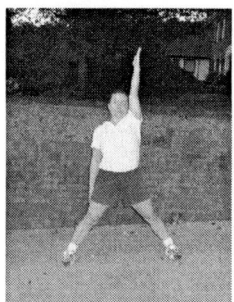 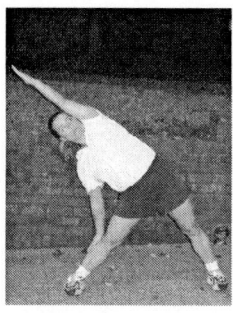

9) The only direction we have not stretched the back with the previous stretches is called lateral flexion of the spine, which is a side stretch. Standing with your feet parallel and in a wide stance, bring the right arm up by your ear and let the left arm be down on the outside of the left leg. Inhale, bringing your arm up as high as you can. Then exhale and stretch directly to the right side. Do not bend forward at the waist, do not look down at your foot, but keep your eyes straight ahead and stretch to the side. This stretch should feel very good and have no strain. Keep reaching up with your right arm and keep the arm to your right ear. After at least five deep breaths, inhale and come back to center, still stretching up as you change arms. The left arm is now up by the left ear and the right arm is hanging to the outside of the right leg. Inhale, lift up with the arm and exhale into a side bend to the left. Keep that ear to the arm and keep stretching upward with the arm. Allow the spine to stretch in a direction that we often miss. After five deep breaths, inhale up to center, exhale and relax.

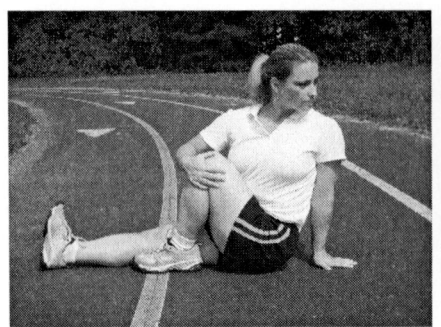 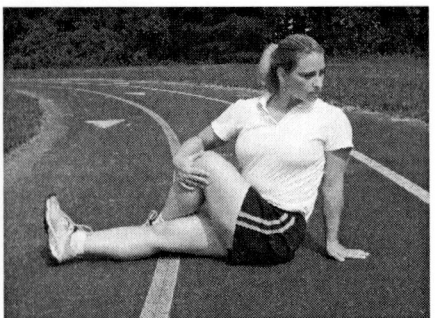

10) Spinal twist. Sit with one leg extended, bend one knee into the chest and place the foot on the floor in one of two ways for the bent knee. Either, the foot of the bent knee can be placed next to the extended leg on the outside or, you can cross the bent leg over and place the foot flat on the ground to the inside of the extended leg. This will add a stretch to the legs. Extend one leg, bend the other knee and place the foot of the bent leg on the floor in one of the variations. Hold the knee of the bent leg with the opposite hand. Next, place the hand of the bent leg directly behind your back in line with the spine with the palm flat on the ground. Look over the shoulder of the hand that is down. Keep your spine straight and with each exhale continue to look further over that shoulder. With each inhale, try to straighten the spine even more. This is a lateral stretch for the spine.

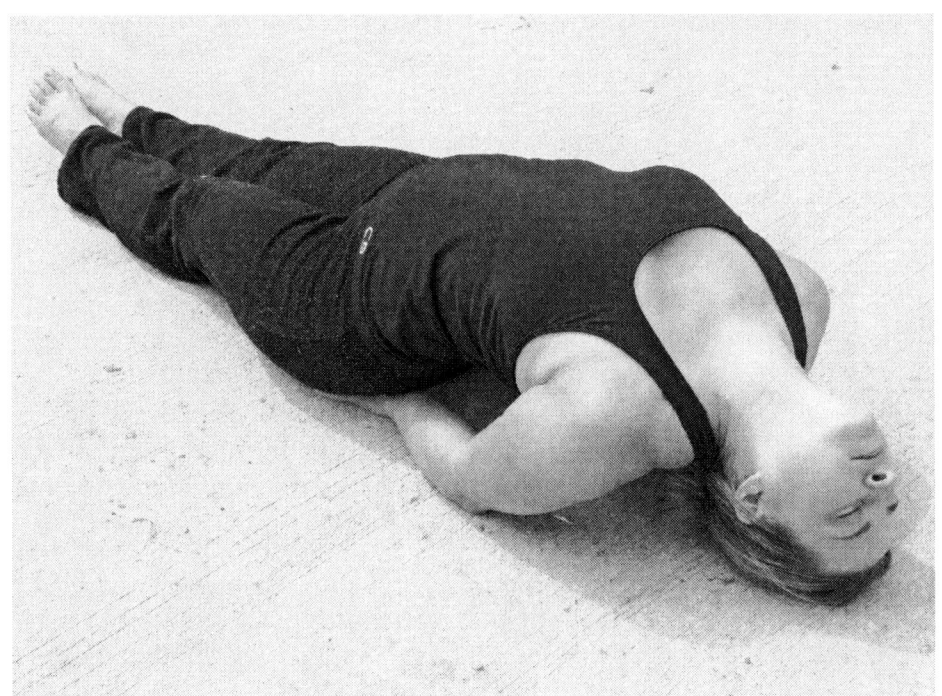

Chest

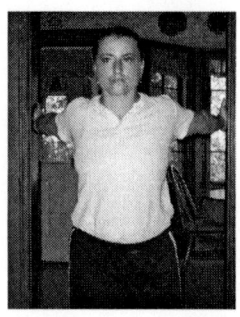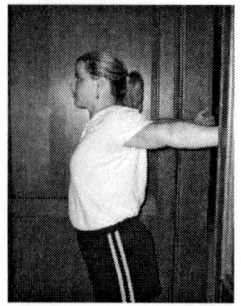

1) The doorway stretch-my personal favorite! If I could pick a single stretch that every client of mine needs, it would be this one. It is simple, extremely effective, and can be done in any setting that has a wall or a doorway. First, the two-handed doorway stretch.

Place both palms on each side of the doorway and come forward until your arms are straight. This stretches the chest and the biceps. For everyone who sits at a desk or at a computer, this one is for you! For everyone else, this is also meant for you because everybody needs to open their chest more. If your chest were more open, you would not have as much pain in your upper back as most people tend to have. You get the point of how important I feel this stretch is...now put it into practice daily, hourly, seriously.

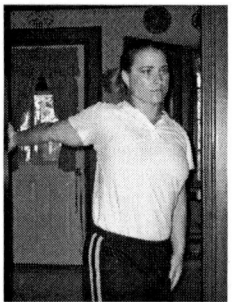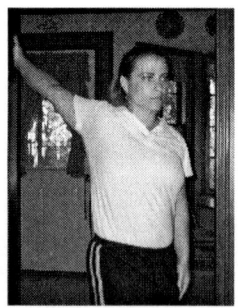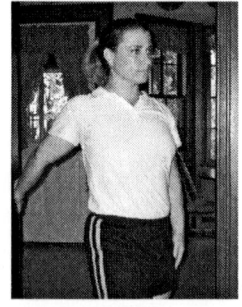

2) The one arm doorway stretch. Place the palm of one hand on the side of the door or wall and walk forward until your feel the stretch in the chest and bicep. When the hand is parallel to the chest you are stretching the entire general area of the chest mostly from the center. When you bring the hand up toward your head you are stretching the lower part of the chest. When you lower your hand to hip level and stretch, you are targeting the upper part of the chest. Keep the breathing fluid and deep and hold these stretches at least five deep breaths.

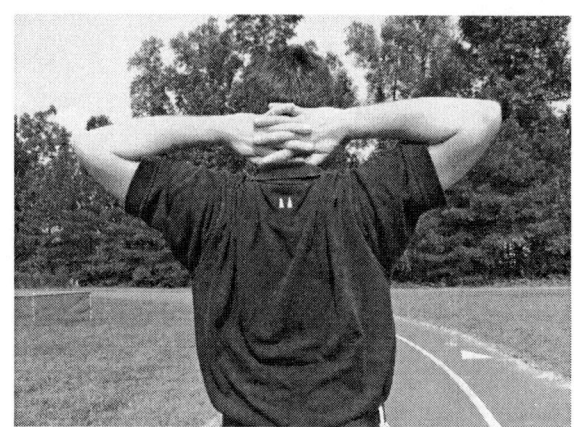

3) Place the hands behind your head and interlace the fingers. Keeping the head up, try to pull the elbows back toward each other. Breathe deeply and let the chest open.

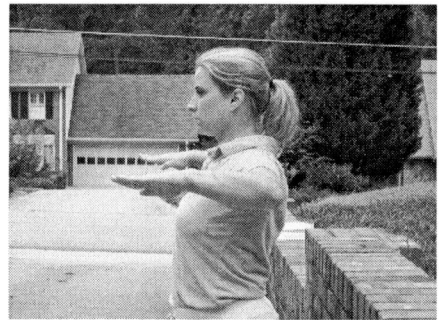 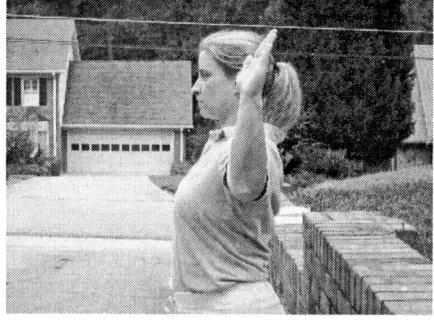

4) To open the chest, this movement is very effective and very basic. It is highly recommended to do right after cycling, running, or kickboxing type of movements. This can be done while walking on your cool down. Place the arms out to the side at a ninety-degree angle with the palms facing the ground. Keeping the elbows in the same place, lift the palms up to face straight ahead-the same direction as your head and the fingertips face upward to the sky. Slowly, rhythmically lift and lower the palms, keeping the elbows still. Feel how the chest and the back work together to open the chest up. If you cycle or are doing an exercise where your chest is rounded, this stretch is really important to do immediately following the exercise so that you don't get in a habit of training your chest to stay in a rounded position.

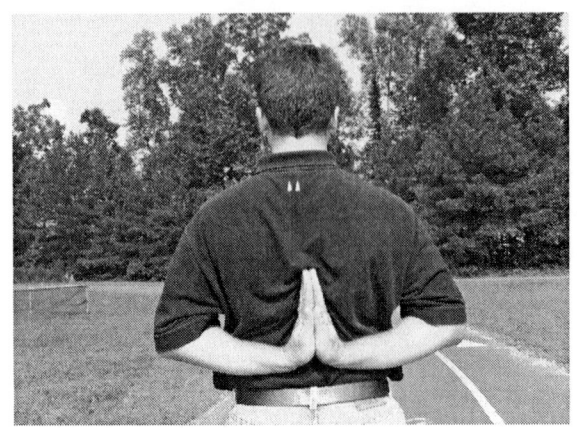

6) "Reverse Prayer" position. This looks incredibly difficult, but for many people this comes easily and naturally. It depends on your body type. For me it is very hard, but for my mother it comes easily. She has longer arms than I do! Start by bringing your hands behind your back and touching your fingertips together. When your fingertips are lined up together, bring the palms inward toward your back and try to bring the pinky side of your palms to the back having the fingertips facing upward. Like I said, for some people this is pretty easy to do and for others it's very difficult but try it, practice it, and play with it a little. You may really surprise yourself. If you can hold this, really focus on how your chest opens up and lift your head up. Breathe deep!

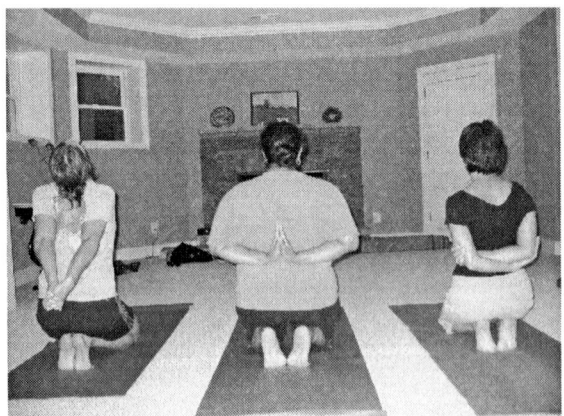

7) If the reverse prayer position is too difficult, try to clasp your hands behind your back. Another variation is to try to grab your arms or elbows behind the back. All three are highly effective.

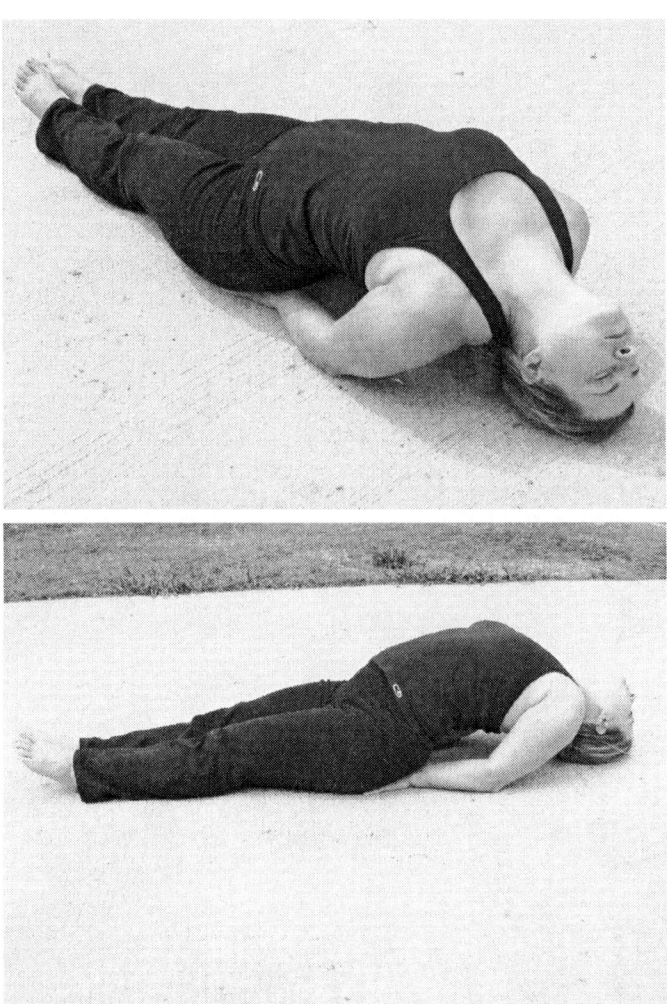

8) The "fish" pose. Lie on your back and place your palms facing down underneath your bottom. Then, sit up on your forearms with your hands still under your bottom. Once you're sitting up, try to place the top of your head on the ground. The chest and back are off the ground and lifting up, the throat is open and getting a really nice stretch, as is the chest. The head is comfortable on the ground. Breathe at least five deep breaths here and then lift the head to come out of it. Lift the head up and then lie down on your back. Finally, remove your hands from under your bottom.

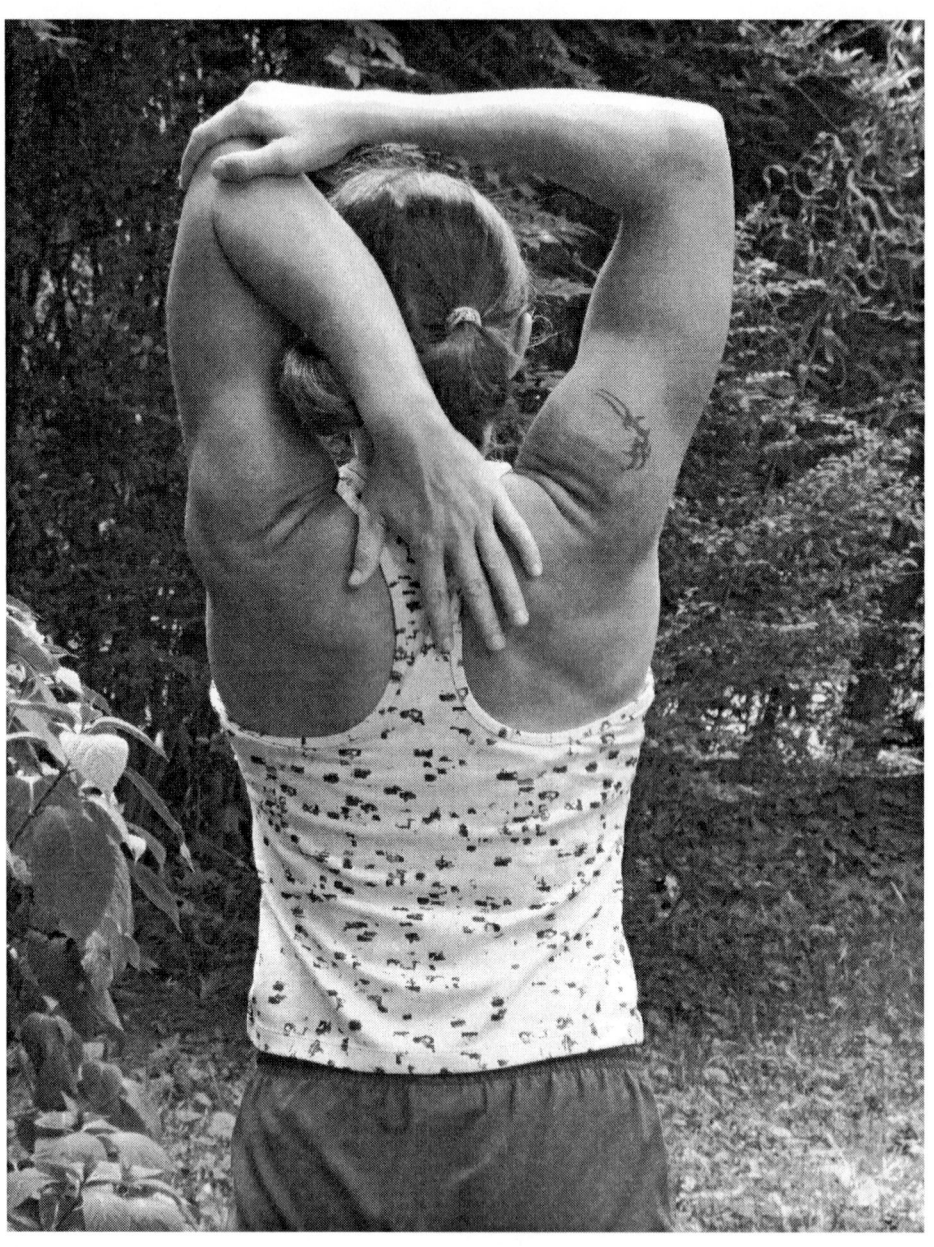

Arms

Biceps:

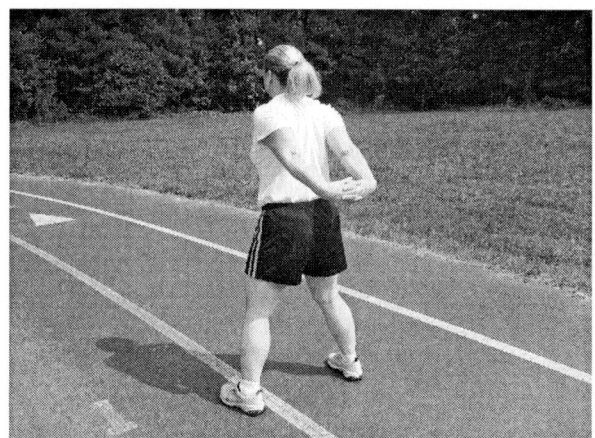

1) Standing with feet wide and parallel, clasp your hands behind your back. Keep your arms straight. As your hands are clasped together, try to lift the arms as high as you can behind your back. This stretches the biceps. Hold this stretch at least five deep breaths.

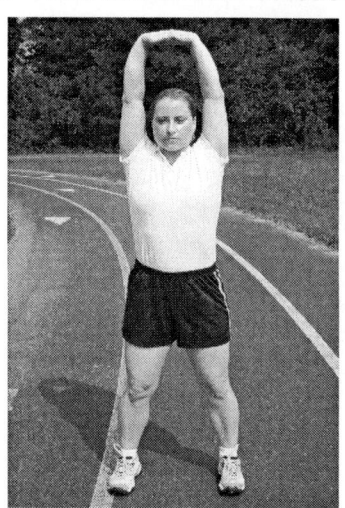

2) Standing in the same position, bring your arms straight out in front of you and interlace the fingers this time turn the palms facing outward and lift your arms up over your head. It is a variation of the previous stretch. Keep reaching the arms up as high as you can and breathe deeply.

3) The doorway stretch as listed on page 49 in the Chest section is also a wonderful way to stretch the biceps.

Triceps:

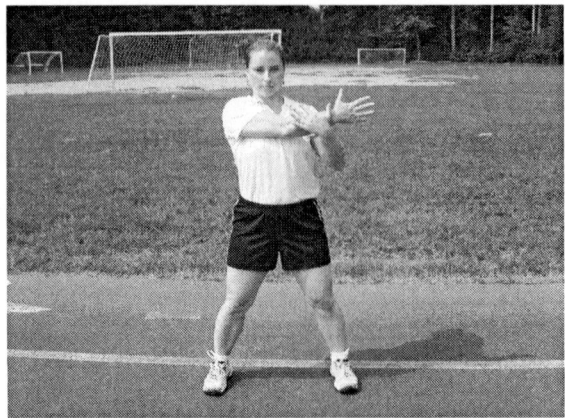

4) Bring one arm across the chest. With the other hand, hold the arm in place-do not place the palm on the elbow but, below the elbow toward the wrist, or above the elbow toward the shoulder. Do this on both sides and hold the stretch at least five deep breaths.

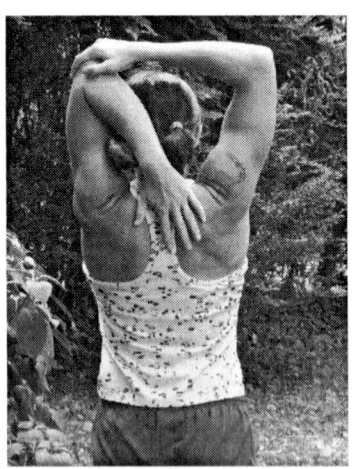

5) Bring one arm up overhead and bend the arm. With the other hand placed on the elbow of the bent arm, assist the stretch by pushing downward. Do not "push" but assist in the stretch. Keep your head up. It is natural to look down when doing this stretch, but try to keep the head at neutral to keep the body in proper alignment. Place the palm of your hand on your back. Change arms and repeat.

Shoulders:

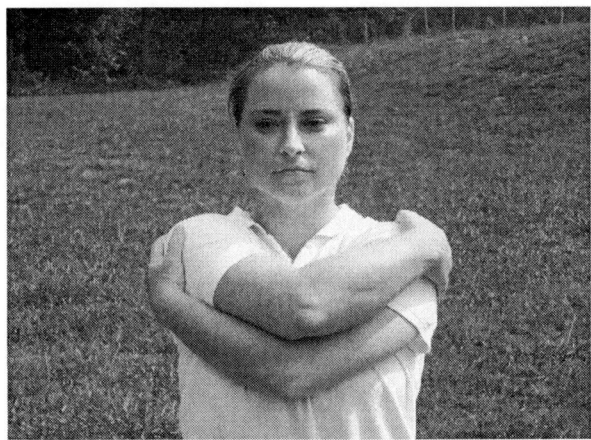

6) Hug yourself! Simply hugging yourself can stretch those shoulders quite nicely and it feels good too!

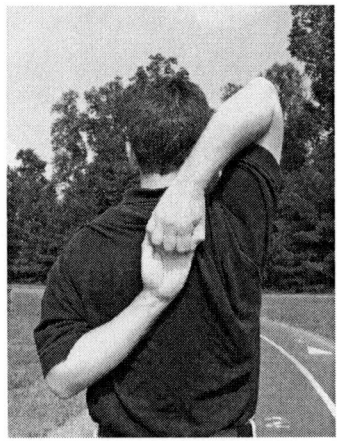

7) Place one hand over your head and bring one hand up from behind your back. Try to get your hands to meet each other in the middle of your back. If the hands touch, try to clasp the fingers to the other hand and hold. Make sure you hold both sides equally-count your breaths. It is very common to be more flexible on one side than the other. However, if there is a big difference, you may want to get that shoulder checked out.

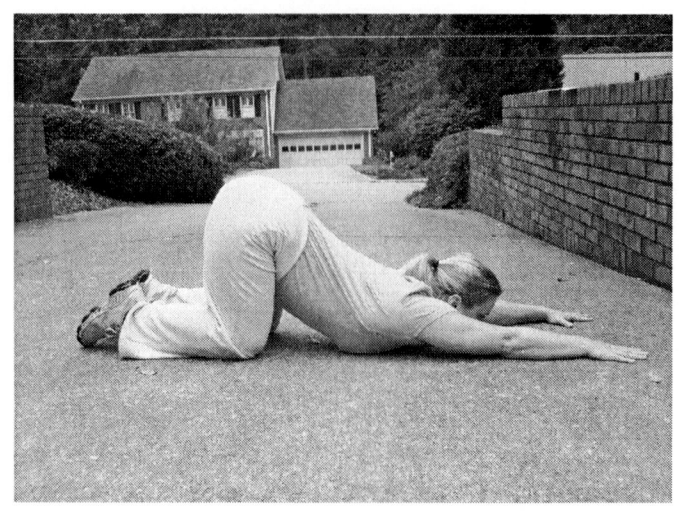

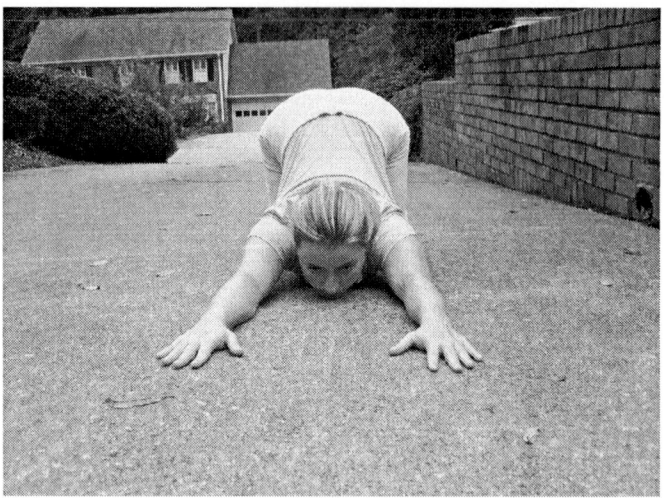

8) "Modified downward facing dog." Start by lying on your stomach. Put the knees on the floor and lift your bottom up as high into the air as possible. The bottom should be in a straight line above your knees. At the same time, place your chin on the floor with your arms stretched out ahead of you and try to get your armpits to touch the ground. This is an excellent shoulder stretch.

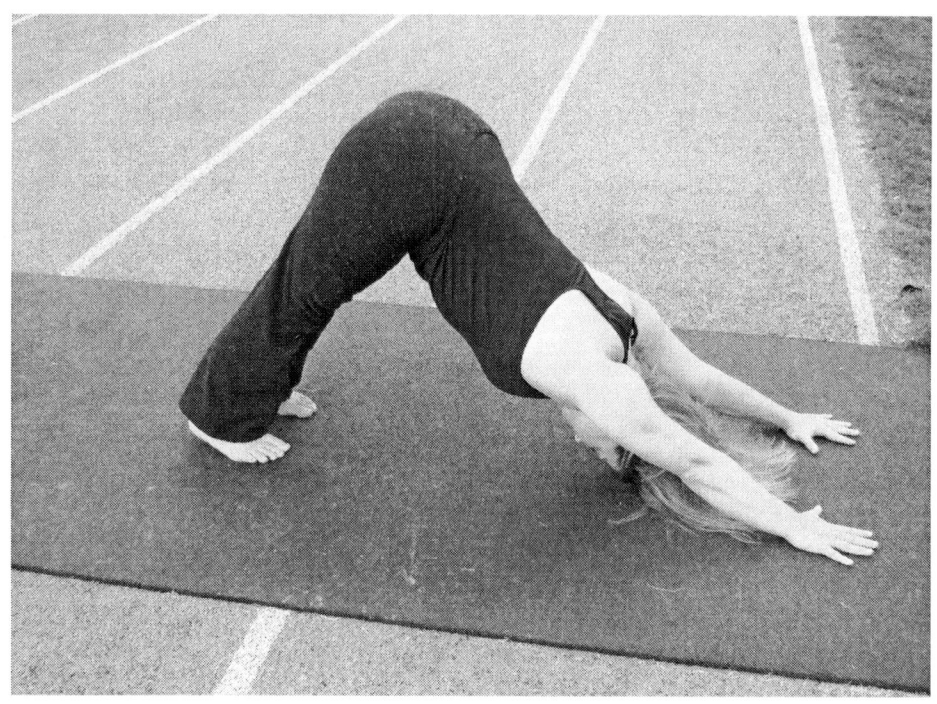

9) "Downward facing dog." You can do the modified first and then come into this stretch.

 Start by putting your palms flat on the ground and instead of being on your knees, lift your bottom up even higher so that your legs straighten and your feet are now on the ground. This looks like a triangle figure-lifting your hips upward like trying to sit on the ceiling. Try to get your heels flat and push back toward your feet. The arms are extended and the head hangs comfortably down. Your armpits still face the floor, but are no longer on the floor. The palms are flat and the middle fingers face straight ahead. The thumbs face each other. A nice way to get into this stretch is to start by bending one leg and then the other. Hold this stretch for at least five deep breaths.

*If you are pregnant, lactating, have high blood pressure, or have glaucoma DO NOT do this stretch!

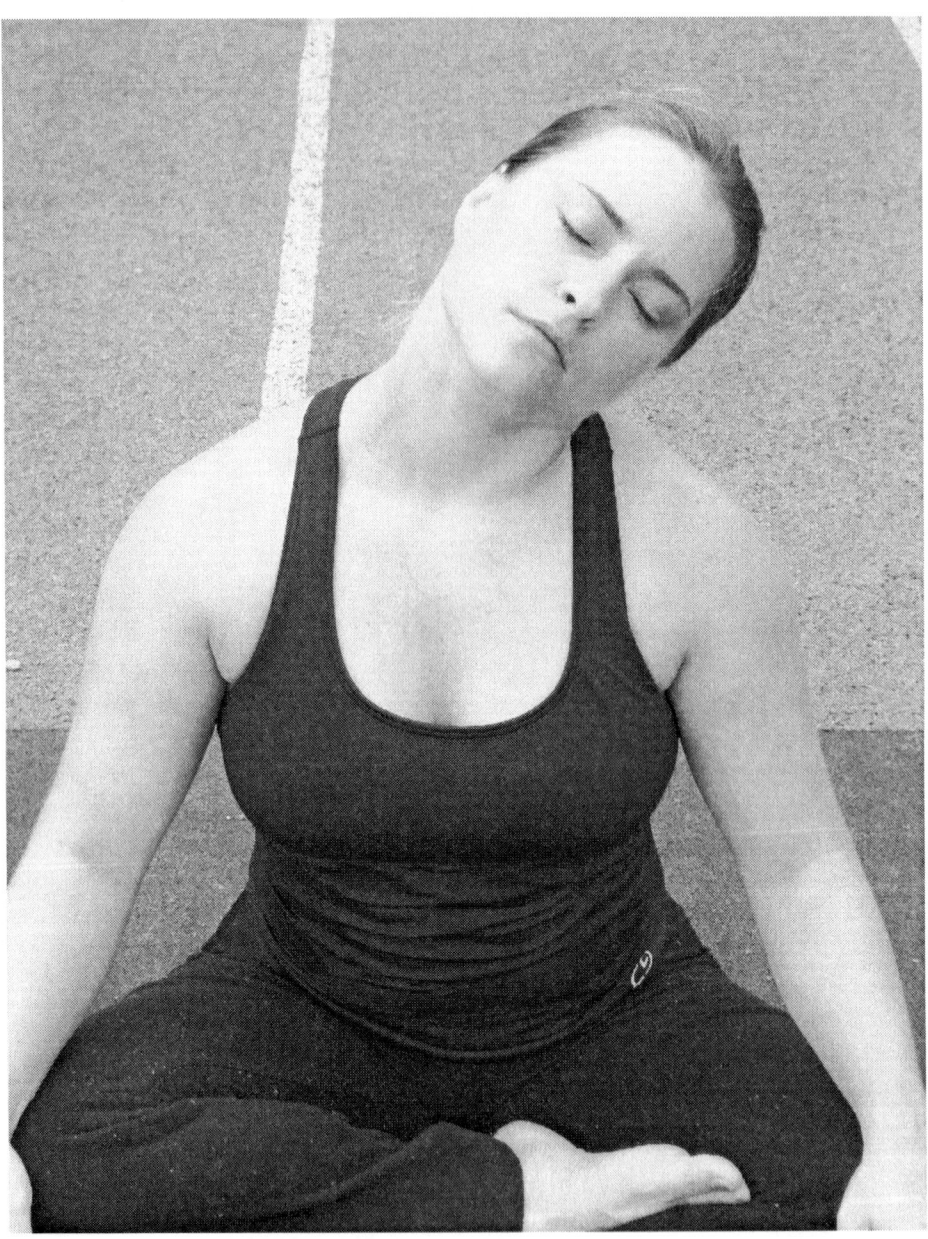

Neck

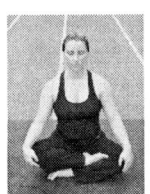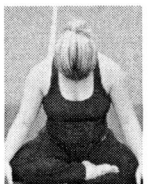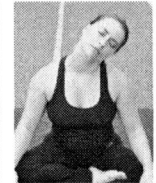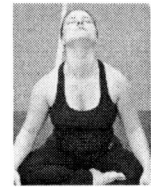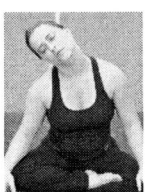

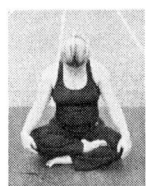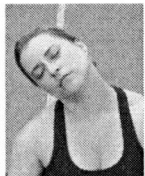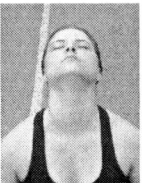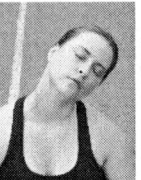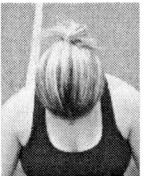

1) First we will start with complete, deep neck circles. It is important to know that some health instruction-related organizations recommend not doing full neck circles. Therefore, if you would rather do *half* neck circles (to the front half-one ear to the shoulder rounding the neck bringing the other ear to the other shoulder) that is an excellent stretch as well. The full neck circles described here are from my tai chi practice. It is done slowly, effectively and has been practiced this way for hundreds of years. I feel comfortable offering this stretch.

The full neck circles must be done slowly, using your breath as a guide. This stretch can be done standing, sitting in a chair, or as I'm doing it, sitting on the ground. If you are standing, keep the legs hip width apart, the knees slightly bent, the spine straight and the shoulders down. If in a chair, all the same apply, except that the knees should be at a ninety-degree angle with feet placed firmly on the floor. When sitting on the ground it is comfortable to sit in "easy position". The legs are crossed, but not over each other. So, both knees are bent and on the ground. One leg is in front of the other leg, but not spread apart. You can sit crossed legged, or with one leg crossed on top of the other. Sit in a way that you can keep your spine straight and you are comfortable.

Begin with your shoulders down, the spine straight, and the head in neutral - meaning that the chin is in line with the sternum/center line of the body. Gently bring the chin down to the front of the chest with an exhale. Begin circling the neck to one side moving very slowly. The trick here is the breathing. The first half of the neck circle is done on the inhale - moving your neck slowly as you inhale a full breath. As the neck gets to the back, continue with the circle, but exhale until the chin arrives at the front of the chest. When you have completed one full circle, CHANGE DIRECTIONS! The neck now circles the opposite direction, still on the inhale for the first half and on the exhale as you complete the circle. Keep the breathing fluid, full and smooth and use your breath as a guide in your speed.

This should be done very slowly, rhythmically, and most importantly...easily. This should not cause any pain or discomfort. If it does, discontinue this movement and stick with half circles, skipping the backward half of the circle.

It is nice to do at least three rounds of these circles. When you feel you've stretched enough, come up from the center. When the chin is down into the chest, simply lift the head with a nice inhale and as you exhale, open your mouth and let out a sigh or vocalized breath on the exhale. This just makes the stretch end really fluidly and pleasantly.

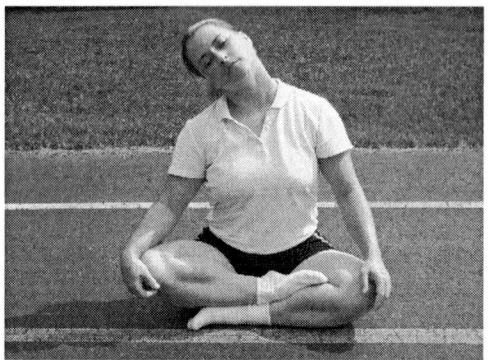

2) Start in the same position that you were in for neck circles (i.e. standing, sitting or sitting comfortably on the ground). The spine is straight and the shoulders are down-not holding any tension and NOT rising up to greet the chin. We often try to increase the stretch, not realizing that we are doing it, and that actually decreases the neck's full range of motion.

Simply bring your right ear down toward the right shoulder. DO NOT LIFT THE SHOULDER TO MEET THE EAR!!!

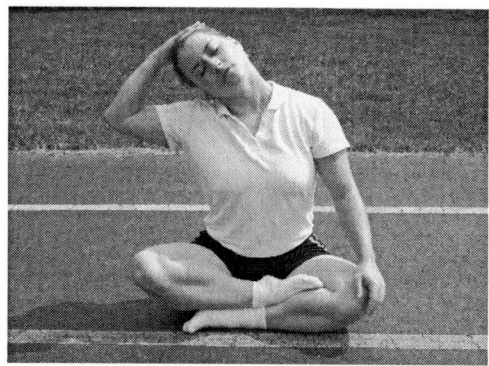

3) To add to this stretch, place the palm of your hand on top of the head and gently assist the neck to stretch a little bit further. Do not yank or pull, and be sure to move very slowly and easily.

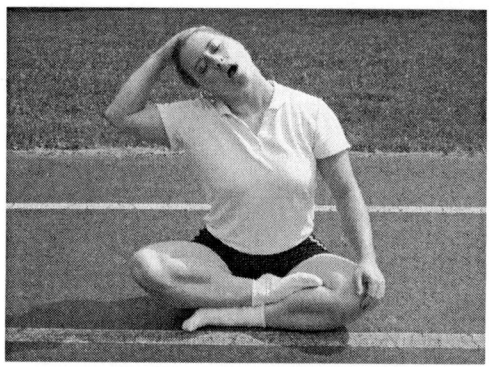

4) To further add to this stretch, simply open your mouth. In this side neck stretch we are stretching our scalene muscles. When we open our mouths it increases both the scalene stretch and the SCM (Sternocleidomastoid-coming from the collar bone to up behind the jaw). Open the mouth wide enough that you feel the stretch coming all the way up into the jaw, but not so wide that you are creating more tension. It's a gentle, calm opening and you will really enjoy this stretch if you move this way. It really does release a lot of tension!

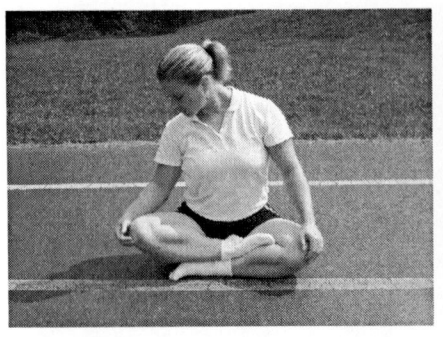 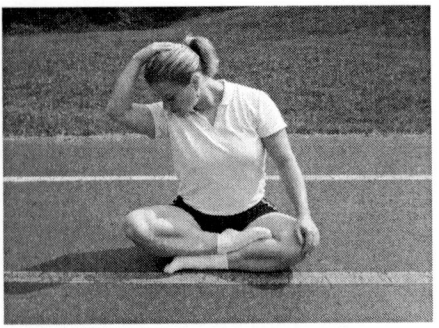

5) Gently, close the mouth and turn your head toward your knee. Your chin and head should be about forty-five degrees from your centerline (the imaginary plane separating your left and right halves) and from the sideline (the plane separating your front and back halves). Simply look down toward your knee if you're sitting in easy position or past your legs if you're sitting in a chair or standing. Bring the chin down and forward in the direction of the chest, but a bit more forward so you can better stretch the cervical spine (vertebrae in the neck). Assist this stretch by placing the palm of the hand on the head and *very gently* add to the stretch. The left hand assists when the chin is facing the left shoulder, and the right hand assists when the chin is facing over the right side. This stretch should stretch the back half of the neck.

*Be sure to do all of these stretches equally on both sides. Try to count your breath so that one side will not be stretched longer than the other.

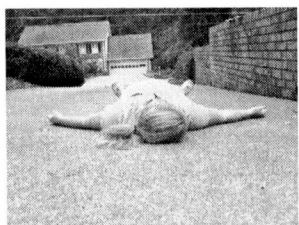 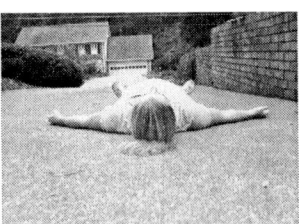 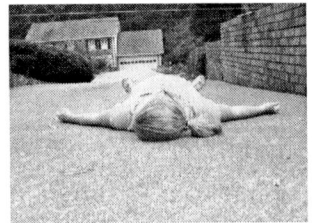

6) Lie down on your back in relaxed position. Your legs are wide, your feet fall out to each side, your arms are out to the side, and your palms face up. Your head starts in neutral and then slowly turns to one side completely - trying to get your ear to the ground. Slowly, turn your head the other direction and do the same thing. This should be done very easily and very often. When you've stretched both sides, bring the neck back to center/neutral and relax.

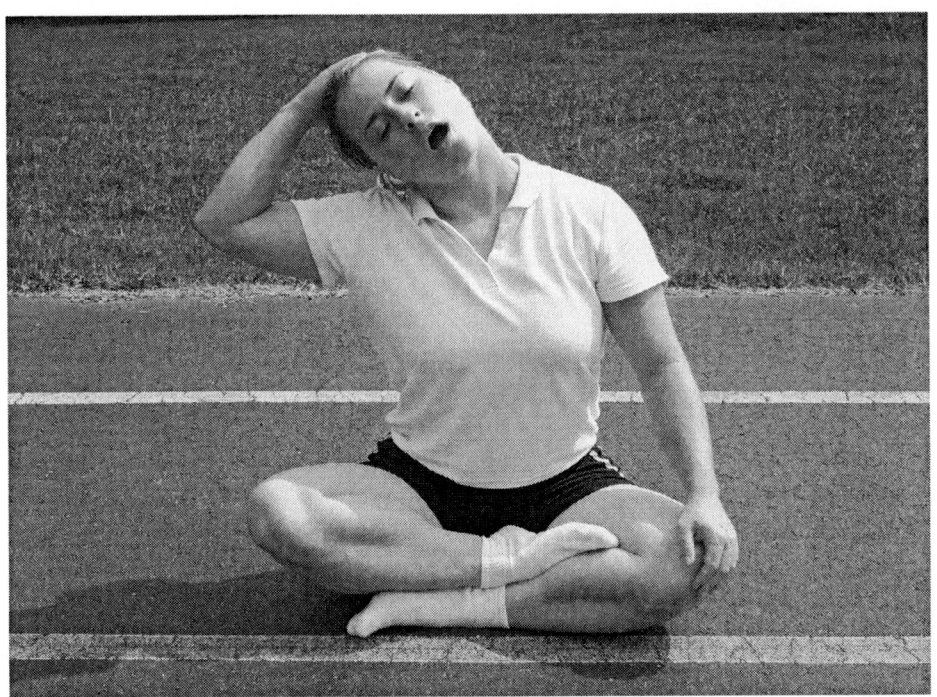

Jaws

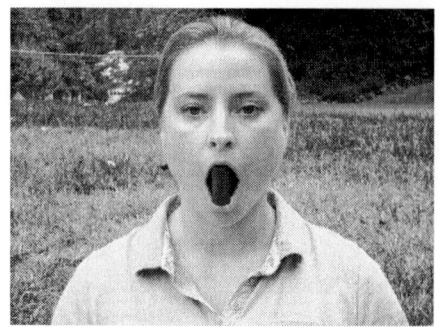 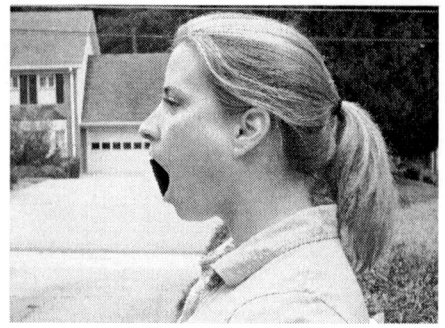

1) There is a wonderfully simple stretch to practice if you have issues with your jaws such as TMJ dysfunction, grinding or clenching of the teeth. The tool you need is a cork, like one from a wine bottle, but any cork will do. (This does not mean I am suggesting drinking wine). Take the cork and place it long ways between the top and bottom teeth. The jaw muscles will relax almost immediately, but try to hold this for at least a minute or two. It's great when you're in traffic and stressed, to just put a cork in your mouth and let it relax. Don't feel like you have to bite/clamp down into the cork, but it is a soft material so it's easy on the teeth. It will probably make you drool a bit, but it's well worth it!

2) See the neck stretch number 4 on page 61.

Relaxation:

 Once you have finished stretching, you can either take a few minutes to relax then, or wait until you're in your bed ready to go to sleep. If you chose to relax following exercise, cool down and stretch first. Then simply lie down and close your eyes. You need only a minimum of five minutes to let the exercise absorb into muscle memory and your body/mind to relax. A good position is to lie on your back with your palms facing up and arms about 45 degrees from the body. Let your feet fall out to each side and allow your legs to be wider than your hips. Turn your head from one side to the other and back to middle to stretch the neck. Then, wiggle your fingers and your toes and adjust your body to a comfortable position. Tuck your bottom under slightly and allow your low back to sink into the ground. If it's uncomfortable to lie flat on your back, you can place a pillow under your knees, or lie on your side. You can simply go through the body from toes to head or vice versa tightening the muscle group and then relaxing the muscle group. Example: curl the toes under and then release them. Clench the calve muscles and then relax them. Move your way up the legs, the back, the chest, the shoulders, the arms, the hands (make a fist and release) and the face muscles. Once the muscles are relaxed, focus on your breath by slowing it down. Make each inhale and exhale long and smooth. Let the breath become silent and fluid. As for breathing for relaxation, it is best to inhale through the nostrils and exhale through the mouth. Let your body relax into each breath. To add to this you can do what I call "gratitude breathing" which is where each inhale you think of something positive and healthy; a key word or phrase. On the exhale, release something that no longer serves a healthy purpose. Keep the thoughts and words simple. Use this as a way to allow the breath to direct you into a calm, healthy state of being.

Give yourself praise for a job well done with your exercise, your stretching, and the fact that you've taken time out to relax and honor your experience. To get up, slowly wiggle your fingers and toes, reach your arms up over your head, and stretch the body from head to toe. Bend the knees and roll to the right side of the body because it follows the blood flow from the heart *(unless you are pregnant or lactating then roll to your left side) Help yourself up to a seated position and remain in a seated position for a few more breaths. When you're ready, open your eyes and continue with your day!

If you chose to wait until you're ready for bed, the relaxation session should be longer and lead you into sleep. Lie down in your bed in a very comfortable position on your back. You can place a pillow under your knees, and one under your neck if you like, or you can lie flat. You want your feet to be wider than your hips, your palms about 45 degrees from your torso and your palms facing up. As with the quicker relaxation, you want to move your head all the way to one side and all the way to the other before resting in the center. If you choose, you can go through the muscle tensing and releasing exercise or you can follow this simple meditation.

It does not have to be in this order nor it does it have to be this specific. This is simply an example of what I use and what I have learned from my yoga teacher when we relax.

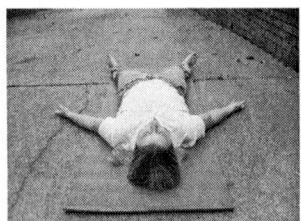 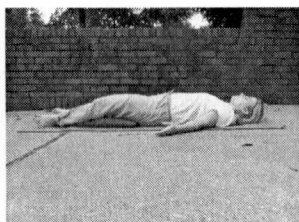 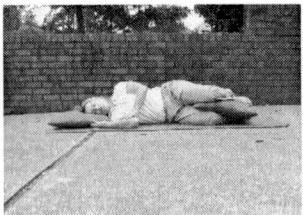

Start with your feet and repeat in your head:

Relax my feet.... my feet are relaxing...my feet are relaxed.

Relax my calves...my calves are relaxing...my calves are relaxed.

Relax my thighs...my thighs are relaxing...my thighs are relaxed.

Relax my hips and low back...my hips and low back are relaxing...my hips and low back are relaxed.

Relax my entire back...my back is relaxing...my back is relaxed.

Relax my stomach...my stomach is relaxing...my stomach is relaxed.

Relax my chest...my chest is relaxing...my chest is relaxed.

Relax my arms...my arms are relaxing...my arms are relaxed.

Relax my hands...my hands are relaxing...my hands are relaxed.

Relax my neck...my neck is relaxing...my neck is relaxed.

Relax my head/scalp...my head is relaxing...my head is relaxed.

Relax my face...relax my eyes, relax my eyebrows, relax my nose, relax my lips, relax my jaws, relax my chin...my face is relaxing, my face is relaxed.

Relax my entire body...my entire body is relaxing...my entire body is relaxed.

Relax my brain...my brain is relaxing...my brain is relaxed.

Relax my heart...my heart is relaxing...my heart is relaxed.

Relax my lungs...my lungs are relaxing...my lungs are relaxed.

Relax all vital organs...all vital organs are relaxing...all vital organs are relaxed.

Relax my entire being...my entire being is relaxing...my entire being is relaxed

Once you have gone through your entire body, simply allow yourself to be a witness to your breathing, your body, your calm, beautiful self-holding no stress. Just watch yourself and follow your breathing. Inhale bringing in peace and calm with every breath into your being, and releasing all tension and stress on the exhale. Continue to feel the exchange of energy through your breathing and when you're ready, allow yourself to drift off to a nice, deep, complete sleep for the night. Enjoy the freedom you feel in being calm and centered. Take advantage of how you feel and re-create this feeling every night. Remember...you can never be too relaxed!

About the Author

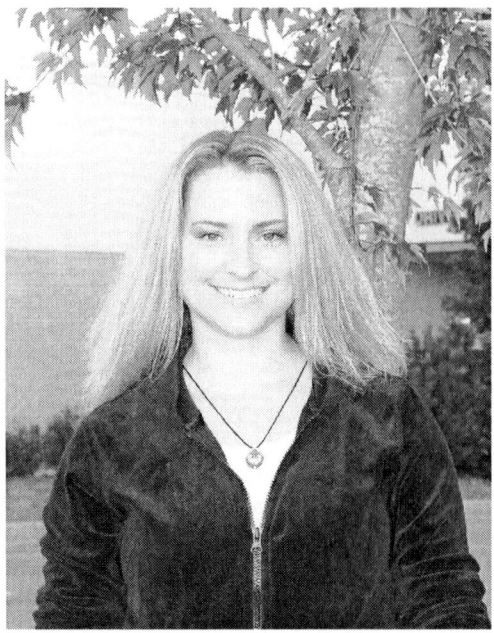

Emily Smith holds a BS in Exercise Science and Wellness from Jacksonville State University

Minor in Nutrition/Dietetics

A Nationally Certified Clinical/Neuromuscular therapist from the Atlanta School of Massage

A Universal Yoga Teacher in Sivananda Yoga

A Usui Reiki/Karuna Ki Master

A Doctor Vodder graduate for Manual Lymph Drainage and Combined Decongestive Therapy

Since graduating college in 1998 she has served as an aerobic director, a yoga instructor, a martial art/tai chi practitioner, head of the health and physical education department for a high school and currently is in private practice for a variety of healing work.

Http://www.myspace.com/vishnugirl

Acknowledgements

A very special thank you to Ivan Ruyle for putting this entire text together along with me.

Thank you: Larry Pepper, Janice St Hilaire, Courtney Raiser, Sandy Glover and all of my clients for making me realize the value of putting this together.

Edited by: Tim Holmes

Heather Hale for proofing this text

Joanna Colabello-Sole for the nondisclosure agreement/legal advice

Dattatreya For being my yoga teacher and an incredible inspiration

Kris Bush: Sales/marketing

My family: Peg Smith, Bradley and Emilie Smith, Margaret Oliva, Gretchen Studdard, James Studdard and the late Jim Smith for unending support and love.

All of my angels, guides and divine graces for infusing me with these ideas and inspirations.

Photos by: Ivan Ruyle, Patty Jervey, Emily Smith

Head Shot: Jill Kostrinsky

Photos of: Emily Smith, Heather Hale, Mikhail Raznobriadsev, Ivan Ruyle, Julia Ripley, Ziba Malek and Jyoti Patel.

Cover Design by Ivan Ruyle